The International L

DYNAMIC SOCIAL RESEARCH

Founded by C. K. Ogden

The International Library of Psychology

SOCIAL PSYCHOLOGY
In 7 Volumes

DYNAMIC SOCIAL RESEARCH

JOHN J HADER AND EDUARD C LINDEMAN

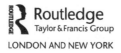

Routledge
Taylor & Francis Group

LONDON AND NEW YORK

First published in 1933 by
Routledge, Trench, Trubner & Co., Ltd.
2 Park Square, Milton Park, Abingdon, Oxfordshire OX14 4RN
711 Third Avenue, New York, NY 10017

First issued in paperback 2014

Routledge is an imprint of the Taylor and Francis Group, an informa business

British Library Cataloguing in Publication Data
A CIP catalogue record for this book
is available from the British Library

Dynamic Social Research
ISBN 0415-21118-2
Social Psychology: 7 Volumes
ISBN 0415-21134-4
The International Library of Psychology: 204 Volumes
ISBN 0415-19132-7

ISBN 13: 978-1-138-87574-6 (pbk)
ISBN 13: 978-0-415-21118-5 (hbk)

To

HERBERT CROLY

WHO FURNISHED THE INITIAL INSIGHTS
AND ENCOURAGEMENTS FOR OUR ATTEMPT
TO RE-EVALUATE SOCIAL RESEARCH

CONTENTS

PART ONE

CONFRONTING THE SOCIAL PROBLEM

PART TWO

DEVELOPING A SOCIAL PHILOSOPHY

PART THREE

CLARIFYING SOCIAL METHODOLOGY

PREFACE

THE study upon which this volume is based was conducted under the auspices of *The Inquiry*, an organization devoted to the analysis and improvement of conference methods. The project began as a fact-finding investigation directed toward newer phases of industrial management, particularly managerial instruments in which both employees and employers participated. (Such instruments are usually called 'employee representation' or 'company unions.') We soon realized that significant facts of the variety which we desired were not readily available and that ordinary devices of social research were not suitable for our purposes. Consequently, the study developed in the direction of exploration with newer research techniques and it finally became a project in research method rather than a conventional fact-finding inquiry.

We have chosen to name the published result of our study *Dynamic Social Research* and this title calls for a brief explanation. Our chief purpose in using the adjective 'dynamic' is to indicate our belief that social research should somehow be usable as an implement of social change. In the second place we hold the conviction that social change will in the future be brought about primarily through the use of collective agencies, and that an understanding of these functional groups (collective instruments of control) becomes imperative for our time. And, in the third place, we believe that social research may become dynamic only when investigators are prepared to divest themselves of certain naïve preconceptions concerning so-called objectivity, disinterestedness, and value. Dynamic social research should, therefore, include that variety of fact-finding which is designed to implement social change; which illuminates that area of social relationships which is involved in the operation of functional groups; and which allows for the interpretation of its facts in terms of human purposes, desires, and values as expressed in the research agents.

We are deeply indebted to *The Inquiry* for placing at our disposal its extensive accumulation of data relating to conference methods, for the collaboration of its workers, and especially for allowing us to alter the character of the study from one of fact-finding to methodological exploration while it remained under their supervision. And, we are also grateful to numerous persons in at least five important industries who gave freely of their time and energy on our behalf; many of these must have known from the outset that our highly theoretical preoccupations could not be easily transformed into utility for them but they continued to aid us by contributing to our co-operative projects.

JOHN J. HADER and
EDUARD C. LINDEMAN.

NEW YORK,
March 1933.

Dynamic Social Research

INTRODUCTION

"The time ought to come when no one be judged an educated man or woman who does not have insight into the basic forces of industrial and urban civilization"—JOHN DEWEY.

IN one of the less important offices of a giant corporation a meeting is being held. Here are gathered together mechanics, artisans, and semi-technical craftsmen, and representatives of the management of the industry. The former have been elected as representatives by their fellow-workers and have come to discuss a problem which affects them. Altogether there are fourteen persons in the room, eight employees and six representatives of management; these fourteen persons constitute a joint committee which operates as a part of a general plan of employee representation. Viewed from above this committee session might appear thus :

Chairman of the   Presiding
Employee Group :   Chairman : a representative of Management
    [1]   [1]

  Employee Representatives :   Management Representatives :
[2] [3] [4] [5] [6] [7] [8]   [2] [3] [4] [5] [6]

One of the employees has expressed a grievance, and he is attempting to convey to those present something of the thought and feeling of his fellow-workers. He . . .

A   1

but the reader may as well follow the dialogue as it actually occurred :

Employee Representative 1 (Chairman of the employees' group) : " The employees' committee understands that there has been some unwarranted and unofficial pressure put on some of the newer boys on installation work for producing quantity."

Employee Representative 2 : " When some of the newer boys get their installer's kits, they are put under considerable pressure to get quantity and I think that in these cases quality is being sacrificed for speed. It seems to me that the boys are started with the wrong point of view, if they are told that they have to complete the average installation job in one and a half hours. Some of us older men feel these boys are not getting a fair break."

Management Chairman : " On the contrary, I think just the reverse is true. We lay every emphasis on a good quality construction job and no urge for speed is made at all. As a matter of fact our last check inspection for quality showed a falling off. Management is responsible for the action of the supervisors and I guess there has been some misunderstanding on the part of certain foremen as to what we want. I am certainly glad to get this comment so that we can correct any misunderstanding. We want quality first and time as good as we can get it after this."

Employee Representative 2 : " Some customers have said to me ' How many jobs do you have to do in a day ? ' and that looks to me as though installers must give the impression that we are after speed. I don't think it's a good impression to leave with the public and it may lead them to think we are doing a sloppy job."

Management Chairman (Addressing E. R. 2) : " Joe, do you think all the men feel that way about it ? "

Employee Representative 2 : " No—I think the older men have the correct point of view : it's just that some of the newer boys are getting off to a wrong start."

Management Chairman : " Well, I'm glad to get this information. I've already taken it up in some of the foremen meetings, but I'll go further into the matter now."

Employee Representative 2 : " Down on that Packard building job a couple of weeks ago, I had to spend several hours straightening out another man's job which he had done so poorly."

Management Chairman : " I'm glad to see you've got the right point of view."

Employee Representative 1 : " Where do these new fellows get this idea of speed anyway. It can't be at the plant school for they don't teach it there. I don't see where they get it."

(Note.—No attempt was made to answer this question specifically.)

Management Chairman : " We gain nothing by quick installation at the sacrifice of maintenance. Each job we send a maintenance man on afterwards costs us approximately $1.00 ; therefore the spending of an additional $0.50 on producing good-quality installation means a net saving. It also has a good effect on customers, many of whom would condemn a poor or hastily done job. Apparently this applies to about twelve men who were put on since last fall."

Employee Representative 2 : " Yes, those are the men."

Management Chairman : " I'll clear this up definitely when I see the district installation foreman. This situation that you men have presented may be responsible for the falling off in quality which was mentioned before. It's a good idea to bring up the matter and I'll see that it is straightened out. Is there any other business ? "

For the moment we may restrain our critical inclinations with respect to the committee session reported above and regard it merely as a social phenomenon. What took place at this meeting may be described as a series of interactions between persons representing two groups, two points of view, and two interests, and these interactions may be viewed as lines of communication, each line indicating an importance of its own, as in the chart on the following page.

How significant, in reality, is an event of this sort ? If one knew something more or less fundamental concerning this employee's grievance, the chairman's method of dealing with his request, the conclusion reached, the kinds of responses exchanged, et cetera, would this be a part of that industrial " insight " which Professor Dewey believes to be the necessary equipment of an educated person ? How much light, indeed, would such knowledge cast upon the complicated problem of modern business management ?

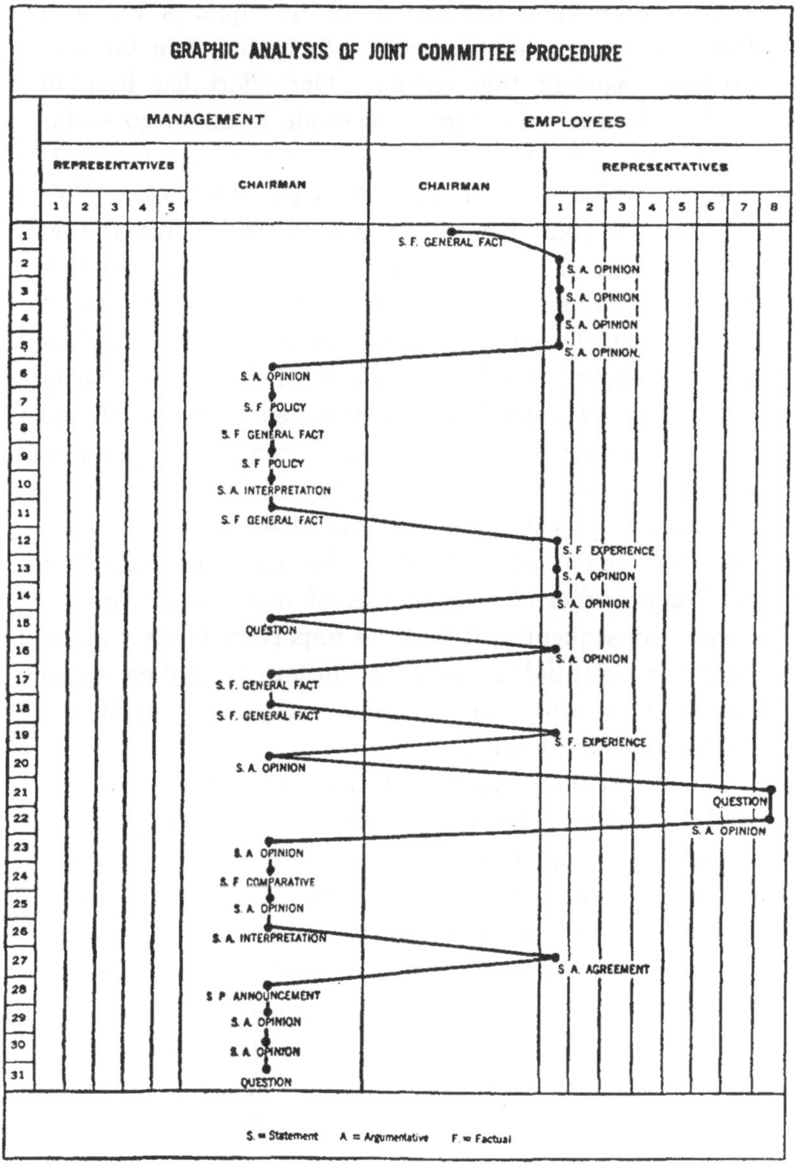
GRAPHIC ANALYSIS OF JOINT COMMITTEE PROCEDURE
MANAGEMENT
EMPLOYEES
REPRESENTATIVES
CHAIRMAN
CHAIRMAN
REPRESENTATIVES
1 2 3 4 5
1 2 3 4 5 6 7 8
1 2 3 4 5 6 7 8 9 10 11 12 13 14 15 16 17 18 19 20 21 22 23 24 25 26 27 28 29 30 31
S. F. GENERAL FACT
S. A. OPINION
S. A. OPINION
S. A. OPINION
S. A. OPINION
S. A. OPINION
S. F. POLICY
S. F. GENERAL FACT
S. F. POLICY
S. A. INTERPRETATION
S. F. GENERAL FACT
S. F. EXPERIENCE
S. A. OPINION
S. A. OPINION
QUESTION
S. A. OPINION
S. F. GENERAL FACT
S. F. GENERAL FACT
S. F. EXPERIENCE
S. A. OPINION
QUESTION
S. A. OPINION
S. A. OPINION
S. F. COMPARATIVE
S. A. OPINION
S. A. INTERPRETATION
S. A. AGREEMENT
S. P. ANNOUNCEMENT
S. A. OPINION
S. A. OPINION
QUESTION
S. = Statement A. = Argumentative F. = Factual

We do not know the answers to these queries, but such clues as we have discovered are to be found in the succeeding pages of this volume. Our effort has been to explore beneath the surface of crude facts, to go so far as our tools would permit into that region of economic process which is essentially human and social. We selected the joint committee in employee representation as our point of departure because we believed that this phase of industrial management offered possibilities of analysis which would not have been so readily realized in other areas. The main business of the world is being conducted by committees or conference groups of one sort or another. Wherever size or complexity prevents a single person from encompassing the total situation ; wherever responsibility needs to be shared or distributed ; wherever man comes to recognize the wastefulness of arbitrary authority, committees of one sort or another arise. Consequently, it becomes important to understand both the potentialities and the limitations of these social instruments which are steadily encroaching upon the authority of individuals.

If interest and opportunity had existed, we might as well have begun to study committees at any point in industrial management, that is, committees of managers, of technicians, arbitration boards, union-management committees, et cetera, et cetera. But, our chief desire was to investigate industry at that point where the interests of employers and employees converge, where the problem of management is primarily the problem of human relations, and the joint committee appeared to offer excellent opportunities for study in this area. When a single unit from the large whole of corporate industry is selected for observation it is, of course, likely that this unit will be over-emphasized and its importance exaggerated. We cannot presume to have escaped this likelihood, but it has been our aim throughout to keep in mind the context of the larger whole. In the backgrounds of our minds were five persistent queries which we were continuously directing toward the joint committee, and we attempted to see these queries in the light of the total situation of which joint committees were merely a part. This total situation may be viewed in terms of the chart below :

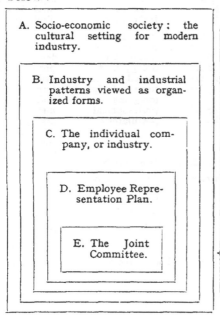

A. Socio-economic society : the cultural setting for modern industry.

B. Industry and industrial patterns viewed as organized forms.

C. The individual company, or industry.

D. Employee Representation Plan.

E. The Joint Committee.

a. The joint committee as structure. (What is it as social form ?)

b. The joint committee as process. (What is it as social process ?)

c. The joint committee as procedure. (What method or procedure does it utilize ?)

d. The joint committee as function. (What problems does it deal with ?)

e. The joint committee as result. (What quality of results does it achieve ?)

Every science is founded upon hypothesis; indeed, there can be no science without hypothetical presuppositions concerning both the reality which is to be investigated and the devices to be utilized for fact-finding purposes. As a consequence of our study of joint committees we have formulated an hypothesis for social research which consists of four major divisions which now become the main parts of this volume; the reader may find it useful to have this hypothesis in mind at the outset, at least in the form of a total inquiry, and the ensuing chart should serve this purpose:

THE TOTAL INQUIRY

1	2	3	4
Confronting the Social Problem :	Evolving a Social Philosophy :	Clarifying Social Methodology :	Experimenting with Social Techniques :
What is a joint committee in industry ? *Why* do joint committees exist ?	How may the problem of the joint committee (as an object of research) be stated in terms of social philosophy ?	How may the problem of social methodology be restated in terms of the foregoing philosophical postulates ?	What techniques and devices are appropriate for utilizing the foregoing hypothesis and method in the discovery of relevant and pertinent facts ?

THE TOTAL AFFIRMATION

The Rise of Employee Representation and Joint Committees in Modern Industry	The committee process consists of : Impulsion	Value and Subjectivity are Involved in all social research.	The available techniques are : Interviewing, Direct Observing,
The Joint Committee as an Instrument of Industrial Management and as an Object for Psycho-social Research.	Circumjacence. Interaction. Emergence.	The research situation is modified by the research purpose.	Participant observing, Case analysis, Statistics, Charting.

PART I

CONFRONTING THE SOCIAL PROBLEM

I. THE RISE AND SIGNIFICANCE OF EMPLOYEE REPRE-
SENTATION IN INDUSTRIAL MANAGEMENT.

II. THE JOINT COMMITTEE AS INSTRUMENT OF INDUSTRIAL
MANAGEMENT AND AS OBJECT FOR PSYCHO-SOCIAL
RESEARCH.

PART ONE

CONFRONTING THE SOCIAL PROBLEM

THE multiplicity of social researches now in process or projected by social scientists furnishes cause for both assurance and misgiving. Our misgivings are, perhaps, more worthy of notice at the moment since scientific optimism tends, in spite of occasional set-backs, to reassert itself ; there lives a persistent hope that science will somehow measure our social phenomena and lead us ultimately toward rational control of events. This is not an unreasonable hope but it is often pursued in unreasonable fashion. Certainly it is not enough, as some social scientists appear to believe, merely to accumulate studies of isolated phenomena ; the sum of parts does not always make a whole. Nor, does the sum of unimportant researches constitute a total of importance. Confronting a social problem represents an act of wholeness before it can become significant as detail. The student who does not know why he has selected *this* rather than *that* problem for his research may produce results useful to some other scientist but he cannot himself behave as a scientist. The problem selected for social research should have relevancy with respect to present and future social experience ; it should be seen as history and as dynamics, in its antecedents as well as in its thrust into the future. Once the problem has been confronted in this manner of the " whole," specialized approaches may proceed so far as the valid tools of research allow.

CHAPTER I

THE RISE AND SIGNIFICANCE OF EMPLOYEE
REPRESENTATION IN INDUSTRIAL MANAGEMENT

" There is no reason why . . . the labour of supplying
society with all the material goods needed for its general
comfort should not become both agreeable and attractive.
There would be no necessity of waiting for the slow action
of evolution in transforming human character, as contemplated
by Spencer. *The result can easily be brought about by the transformation of human institutions* "—LESTER F. WARD, *Applied
Sociology,* p. 336.

DURING and after the War of 1914–18 many thinkers
essayed to reformulate the equation of social progress.
As so often happens in crises, the slow method of improving
individuals, with the hope of finally altering the mass,
was partially abandoned for the fast-moving device of
transforming human institutions. At least three structural
transformations actually followed, and upon a grand
scale : the social institutions of Germany, Italy, and
Russia, were, in varying degrees, reconstituted. (The
above order of names represents at least one of these
degrees of change : Republicanism in Germany, Fascism
in Italy, and Sovietism in Russia may be regarded as a
graded scale in which the Bolshevist revolution symbolizes
the most radical transformation of institutions.)

But in Great Britain and the United States there was
to be, presumably, an overhauling of a less radical
character ; reconstruction in the Anglo-Saxon nations
was designed primarily as an increase in liberalization

rather than as fundamental social change. One heard, during those fateful days when disillusionment led to prophecy and futurism, much about the revamping of our economic institutions, particularly industry itself. These prophecies have thus far remained unfulfilled. Industrial organization, in the United States, is basically what it was before " reconstruction " became a shibboleth. Three precipitates, though not altogether attributable to the war and its ensuing reconstruction, are, however, observable : (a) Trade unions of the type represented by the Amalgamated Clothing Workers Union have fortified their positions, and have proceeded further in the direction of industrial, as distinguished from craft, unionism ; (b) experiments in co-operation, or collaboration, between organized workers and industrial managers, such as the Baltimore and Ohio Railroad project, have been undertaken ; (c) an increasing number of industries have adopted various plans providing for " employee representation " in management. It is this latter movement which constitutes the preoccupation of the present authors.

When employees participate in the management of an industry it may be said that a partial social transformation has been achieved. Heretofore, managers of industries have assumed that their functions and responsibilities existed as entities wholly different from those of employees. Consequently, the " form " of industry, that is, its social structure, was conceived as, and actually became, a closed group (or individual) which shared its functions with no one. (These managerial groups even still contest the right of government to share in control so long as such opposition is fruitful, and only submit to governmental regulation under compulsion.) Many industries, and especially larger units, have now reconstituted their social forms in such manner as to allow for a bipartite structure. Before proceeding in the direction of analysis of employee representation as a new social form, however, it seems advisable to discuss the reasons, rationalizations, and motivations which may be regarded as the basis of its existence.

Why were Employees granted Representation ?

Among the varieties of reasons given, either in oral or written pronouncements, for the rise of employee representation in industry the following may be distinguished :

(1) Employee representation was, and is, regarded by some industrialists as a *panacea* for dealing with so-called " labour problems." This reason rests upon the general assumption that discontent among workers may be channelled off into other forms of activity and need not necessarily lead to disaffection, irregular attendance at work, or more violent outbreaks such as strikes. Once the worker enjoys the privilege of " speaking out " to someone, once his grievances cease to be " bottled up," repressed, and once he realizes that management is not wholly arbitrary he will become a more contented, regular, and loyal employee—so this assumption runs.

(2) Many management groups consider industrial organization to be a form of *benevolent paternalism*. The granting of representation to employees is, obviously, a paternal act. It is analogous to the extension of suffrage by a benevolent ruler, not because subjects demand or deserve

this privilege, but because it is conceived to be " good for them," and because it is likely that their attitude toward the grantor will in consequence be more favourable. Employee representation, both in smaller and more personal companies and in larger, impersonal corporations, is frequently inaugurated as a gift from the employer to the employee. (The paternal ingredient can be readily detected ; wherever paternalism is the chief motivating factor in employee representation one discovers a lingering sentimentality.)

(3) Employee representation plans exist in industries where trade unions once functioned and in some instances was initiated as a *reaction against trade unionism*. There are critics who insist that the whole of employee representation as motivation may be explained on this basis, but we contend that this represents an oversimplification of the situation. Certainly, many employers still adhere to the principle that they will not tolerate or deal with trade unions organized independently and utilizing agents of their own selection in negotiations with management. The majority of such employers entertain a generalized antipathy toward collective action, but they would, in an emergency, accept worker organization " inside " the industry if it promised to forestall " outside " affiliation.

(4) Still other employers, believing in the principle of collective action, and realizing that some form of inter-relation between management and employees in problem solving is essential, have purposefully set up plans of employee representation as the *initial type of association* for their workers. It is entirely probable that many employee representation plans conceived in this manner

would never have come into existence if a suitable form of trade unionism had been available. If one were to distinguish the above types of motivation on the basis of greater or lesser validity, it would seem clear that this latter incentive is far superior to the others, representing as it does a realistic approach to modern industry, plus an experimental attitude.

In addition to the above primary motivations in establishing forms of employee representation it should be admitted that many plans rest upon no clear-cut, basic assumptions ; these have come into existence largely through the influence of imitation. Further, no single source of motivation accounts for any given industry, since the paternalistic attitude persists side by side with a genuine desire to find a social form in which employees may participate with management in directing industrial affairs. In short, precise motivations fitting each case are not discoverable, but the above classifications may be taken to represent a rough approximation of casual factors.

One important situational item has, however, been omitted in the above analysis, namely, the fact that orthodox trade unions themselves may have been responsible for the rise of employee representation. As industry becomes more and more mechanized, it becomes apparent that the meaning of individualized crafts tends to disappear. But, many of the older and well-established trade unions adhere tenaciously to the craft principle of organization regardless of transitions in industrial development. Most employee representation plans allow for organization according to industries, or departments within industries, and this seems to be more in harmony with the actual need. (In certain cases, however, employee representation also provides for recognition of crafts but this recognition is subordinate to a more inclusive conception.)

Employee Representation as a Reflection of Underlying Industrial Conflict.

It may be assumed at the outset that employee representation, no matter what else it includes, constitutes an attempt to deal with the problems of human relationships in industry. The significance of the movement as a whole, therefore, rests upon its capacity to improve these relations, specifically the relations between workers and employers. We are here confronted with a problem which resides primarily in the area of attitude, opinion, philosophy, and social method. If an irrepressible conflict between workers and employers (or, as usually stated, between Capital and Labour) exists, and if, therefore, the relations between these two groups must be conceived as between parties of opposition, any plan for improving these relations will be limited, if not in the end, frustrated.

This is not the place for a comprehensive discussion of the philosophical nature of industrial conflict but enough must be said to clarify the basic hypothesis of the authors. If inescapable conflict exists between the two major parties [1] in industry, workers and employers, the reason

[1] To think of industry as constituted of two parties only is, of course, to oversimplify and falsify the equation. Directly, or indirectly, involved in modern industry are (a) the banks, (b) the stockholders, (c) the managers, (d) the directors, (e) the technologists, (f) the workers, (g) the law, (h) the politician, (i) and the consumer.

must be apparent either in the objective situation itself, or in the minds of those constituting the two groups. And, so long as conflict is inherent in the thinking, the attitudes, and the behaviour of representatives of each group, it is not important to know whether it inheres in the situation or not ; conflict exists if the involved persons believe or think it exists.

Employer, as well as employee, psychology contributes to the conception of inevitable conflict in industry. Leaders of both groups disavow the underlying separation at times, but their pronouncements do not often harmonize with their actions. In crises something approaching implacable class-consciousness and class-division invariably appears. The lines of opposition tend to blur when prosperity seems inclusive, or when an outside danger threatens both sides, but historically the conflict, both as dialectic and as conduct, persists. The Marxian rationale of class-conflict is, therefore, made plausible by the ideology of both workers and employers. Employee representation functions primarily through joint committees in which representatives of management and of workers behave as though they each represented something which is, in its essence and absolutely, divergent, opposed. It is because of this fact that we feel obliged to preface our analysis with a brief critique of the absolutist doctrine of irrepressible conflict. The purpose of this treatment, if not already foreshadowed, is to lay the foundations for an hypothesis which will allow for employee representation, or any other form of experimentation, as a means toward improving human relations in industry.

B

Absolutism versus Relativism.

No adequate historical evidence sufficient to refute the Marxian dogma exists. Certainly, the industrial evolution of the western world contains nothing to warrant the contrary conclusion, namely, that no underlying and fundamental conflict between Capital and Labour is to be found, or having been observed, is now on the way toward resolution. And, obviously, if the conflict formula is believed in sufficiently, it will sooner or later be realized. The result will be different for various regions; here Capital will rise supreme and control the chief sources of power over the total population, and there Labour will play a similar rôle, and a variety of intermediate forms will also appear. Indeed, it may be said that the United States and Russia already represent the opposite poles of this configuration, with Germany, England, Austria, et cetera, standing between. The hope for the future, consequently, lies in some lucky accident which will endow whatever holders of power come to the top with enough humanism to use power wisely. The real problem which underlies this situation is far more significant than anything which can be expressed by the symbols Capitalism and Communism. We are confronted with a world in which Force leading to Power is the central secret. Creative human relations, that is, relations in which differences are assumed to be vital but not absolute, are denied. " A mass of power-persons cannot integrate, can form no organ or *true* society." [1]

[1] *The Rediscovery of America*, by Waldo Frank, p. 79. See Chapters VII and VIII on " The Reign of Power " and " Gods and Cults of Power."

The Marxian formula is historically related to Hegelian absolutism, with, however, a displaced goal. But, Hegelianism, from one point of view at least, was never so absolutistic as are our modern communistic Marxists. Hegel's sequence, his inclusive explanation of event, ran from *thesis*, to *antithesis*, and then to *synthesis*. Modern Marxists, apparently, believe in thesis and antithesis but they forgo synthesis, unless, perchance, they are so naïve as to believe that he who is overcome or annihilated is thereby synthesized. But, synthesis, difficult though it may be, is precisely man's only opportunity for creative conduct. Antithesis, conflict, cannot be eliminated without reducing life to helpless monotony, sterility. But, the function of conflict is to prepare the way for integration. " It is provided in the essence of things," wrote Walt Whitman, " that from any fruition of success, no matter what, shall come forth something to make a greater struggle necessary." But, struggle for what ? If merely for the sake of struggle, and, if merely to wrest power from someone else, where the gain ? Unless, of course, one may be assured that those who have power are, as human beings, inferior to those who strive for it ? But, this is a picture of human nature which cannot possibly fit the facts, no matter what tests of inferiority or superiority are employed. On the other hand, if struggle, conflict, antithesis, is to be utilized for the gradual improvement of human relations, another important choice becomes imperative. The absolutist philosophy of life is easy, probably because it is also simple. One is merely called upon to select a goal sufficiently far off to be quite unrealizable for immediate

time, and then adhere religiously to this goal as the
summum bonum for all people. Fidelity is measured
thenceforth only by one's adhesion to or deviation from
the stated dogma. If the goal does not grow nearer and
clearer, this may be attributed to the stupidity or
mendacity of others. A relativistic philosophy of life, on
the contrary, sets up goals which are realizable ; goals
which one must be prepared to abandon once they have
been reached ; goals which are merely parts of some
larger evolving whole. But, those who do not follow the
absolute way are not overmuch concerned about goals ;
their preoccupation is with means, with methods ; they
aim, first of all, to make sure that whatever means they
utilize are not in essence contrary to their tentative goals.
They will not, for example, presume to create a peaceful
world by means of warfare. Nor will they envisage a
co-operative society built with the tools of force and
coercion.

Those who laboured on behalf of small improvements
here and there within a society admittedly defective were
formerly labelled " reformers " ; they are now called
gradualists in order to distinguish them even more sharply
from those who know what the real end-goal is and are
willing to bring it into existence by quick, revolutionary,
and, if necessary, brutal means. Presumably, the opposite
of a " *gradualist* " is an " *all-or-noneist*," that is, a person
who scorns the small improvement, who regards gradual
change as beneath his dignity, who, in short, can only
play his rôle heroically in a drama where the villain is
unmistakable, and must be annihilated. This state of
mind, more fitting, perhaps, to melodrama than drama,

is, as the psychologists are now insisting, a near relative to other and pathologic forms of grandeur or martyrdom-need. In any case, it is not difficult to prove by simple observations that no individual human being, to say nothing of societies, can live a single day by this philosophy. The principle of growth is not so easily abrogated. We live as "*gradualists*" physiologically, mentally, and socially. Even those social changes, as for example, the French and Russian revolutions, which seem superficially to have arisen suddenly, are in reality parts of a chain in which there has been no break. Change within continuity is Nature's way, at least so far as the evidence of science goes, and we have nothing more reliable to guide us.

The underlying problems of industrial management are not fundamentally altered by even revolutionary changes in political and economic society. The Russian revolution, for example, has not minimized but rather emphasized the need for an understanding between workers, technologists, and managers. There are, without doubt, many more " joint " committees of one sort or another in Soviet than in Czarist Russia. Those who believe that a politico-economic revolution alters at one stroke the entire nature of the social process are, obviously, following a naïve wish. The social forms which now exist in industry, whether in the United States, Germany, or Russia are indicative of what is potential since these are parts of an evolving process which is continuous. An analysis and an understanding of such forms, as *e.g.* joint committees of managers and workers, is essential as background for interpreting the present accurately, and for anticipating the future.

This hypothesis, of course, carries us far beyond the present study. It implies that the whole of modern industry, both as structure and as process, needs to be studied, analysed, and dispassionately interpreted from the point of view of psychology and sociology. A programme of this sort would include studies of trade unions, union-management co-operative plans, employee representation plans, welfare organizations within and without industry, chambers of commerce, manufacturers' associations, et cetera, et cetera. Numerous contributory studies which might readily be fitted into this picture have already been made. Others are now being conducted. But, very often, in the past, studies of industrial structure and process have contributed little or nothing to a real understanding of the important facts. For example, studies have been made of employee representation plans, but usually for the purpose of proclaiming these social forms as evil or good.[1] Likewise, studies of trade unions, conducted for the purpose of revealing " graft," misuse of power, et cetera, furnish almost no insights with which to interpret trade unionism as a modern social phenomenon. The present study, therefore, is merely a beginning, an excursion into an area whose exploration will require life-time journeys.

It will be observed, as the following pages are scrutinized, that the investigators at no time assumed that the objects of their research were static ; on the contrary, they assumed from the outset that joint committees in industry

---

[1] *The Company Union*, by Robert Dunn, is an excellent illustration of this type of study. It probably contains many important facts, but these were gathered for the purpose of proving the iniquity of employee representation.

are changing, evolving units abstracted from a larger whole, and that these units might respond to a multitude of change-inducing stimuli even during the period of study. It was even assumed that the investigators might themselves become stimuli leading to change, and that therefore the committees might not be precisely the same objects at the close of the study as they appeared to be at the beginning. These assumptions, clearly, ran counter to accepted maxims of research ; it is ordinarily believed that research is somehow *pure* in direct proportion to its ability to isolate and control the object of study. But, this is precisely what is impossible in the psycho-social sphere. What is important as psycho-social process is exactly that which is ongoing, continuous. Laboratory experiments may do very well for the purpose of measuring the intensity of human response, the effect of direct stimuli, et cetera, but no amount of artificial laboratory experimentation will ever be able to reproduce the warm realities of actual social situations. It therefore happened that in the present study the investigators candidly took into account the possibility that they might themselves be the instruments of change in the committees under observation, and that attention given to such changes would in itself constitute a valid and integral part of the total project.

The above procedure, however, led to numerous difficulties, some of which were not technical but rather, ethical. For example, once the investigators realized that they were, by reason of their observations, changing the procedures in joint committees, they were obliged to face the question : To what extent were they, as investigators, justified in guiding changes in the direction of what they feel to be improvement ?   This problem arose early in the study and was met in two ways : first, occasional suggestions looking toward improvement of procedures were made to those responsible for the conduct of these joint committees, but only in response to direct inquiries ; second, the investigators refrained from making a definitive criticism and a definitive statement of what they considered good procedures for joint committees until all actual observations were at an end.   It is presupposed that the foregoing statement of the industrial problem, including certain hypothetical inferences regarding psycho-social research to be found here and also scattered throughout remaining chapters, constitute a rationale, if not a logic, for this type of research.

CHAPTER II

THE JOINT COMMITTEE AS INSTRUMENT OF INDUSTRIAL MANAGEMENT AND AS OBJECT FOR PSYCHO-SOCIAL RESEARCH

"Whereas, if the institutional fabric, the community's scheme of life, changes in such a manner as to throw the work-day experience into the foreground of attention and to centre the habitual interest of the people on the immediate material relations of men to the brute actualities, then the interval between the speculative realm of knowledge, on the one hand, and the work-day generalizations of fact, on the other hand, is likely to lessen, and the two ranges of knowledge are likely to converge more or less effectually upon a common ground. When the growth of culture falls into such lines, these two methods the norms of theoretical formulation may presently come to further and fortify one another, and something in the way of science has at least a chance to arise."—*The Place of Science in Modern Civilization*, by THORSTEIN VEBLEN, p. 46.

THE bulk of those words and conceptions which are utilized in discourse concerning industry originated when functional differentiation was still in its beginnings. Consequently it is still difficult to discuss the modern pattern of industrial control without ambiguity, since the terms used often reflect a situation which was far different from that of the present. Thus in the early period of industrial expansion there was no distinction between ownership and management; most industries were, as a matter of fact, the possession of families, and members of the family group were also managers. In partnerships it frequently happened that both parties to the company were skilled in certain aspects of the business; they

25

combined ownership with managership, and often with craftsmanship.

Modern industrial management, as a differentiated function, stands somewhere between the owners and the workers. Its responsibility is to bring about an efficient relationship between materials, processes, and workers, and this responsibility is derived from the owning group. In corporations with large numbers of stockholders this responsibility is still further refined and comes more directly through the channel of boards of directors or trustees who act on behalf of owners. Differentiation of function is not complete and there exist many confusions due to the fact that managers frequently act as if they were owners ; in such instances they direct their attention toward capital, income, and profits. This mixture of functions arises from the nature of management's total responsibility ; in order to achieve an efficient relationship between materials, processes, and workers they must take capital into consideration and to be efficient means to so manage the affairs of the enterprise as to show profits to investors, stockholders. Any given management group which fails to show profits over a given period of time will be replaced by others, since the stockholders are usually insistent upon dividends. In this respect, industrial management is in much the same position as the college football coach ; if he produces a consistently winning team, his tenure of office is secure, but if his teams become habitual losers, he is replaced. On the whole, however, industrial management tends toward more and more differentiation and specialization. Its functions are increasingly derived from the engineering, not the financing, disciplines, and when the term " management " is used hereafter it is intended to carry the connotation of a specialized group of technicians in industry whose primary task is to direct the actual operation of the industry efficiently.

Industrial Management becomes Scientific.

Approximately four decades ago, and largely through the efforts of Frederick W. Taylor, a movement directed toward the application of scientific principles to industrial management began. Hitherto, management principles had been derived primarily from experience ; managers were individuals who possessed knowledge of the practical aspects of industry and who displayed certain traits of leadership. Taylor attempted to demonstrate that the processes and methods by which men manipulated materials were subject to scientific analysis. His work, and that of his colleagues, is now well known and needs no further elaboration except to state that its impact upon the problem of management was startling. It brought new enthusiasms to some and despair to others. On the one hand, it promised new levels of efficiency and profits, and on the other, it foreshadowed something ominous for the worker. The stop-watch and its measurement of the worker's movements, resulting in radical changes in methods of performing work, precipitated a negative reaction. This, of course, usually happens when science necessitates a sharp alteration of habits. The resistance of the workers to scientific management was probably the chief factor in the rise of two succeeding trends, namely, industrial psychology and personnel research.

Scientific management next turned its attention to the problem of the relation between the individual worker and his job. In addition to analysis of the worker's bodily movements attention was now directed toward his personality, his attitudes, habits, aptitudes, et cetera. Studies in fatigue, the effect of rest-periods, the effect of change in occupation, et cetera, were undertaken, all with the goal in mind of discovering how the greatest amount of efficient production could be secured from workers. In short, scientific management devoted itself almost entirely to such applications of science as promised to improve methods of work for utilitarian ends, either by altering the methods themselves, or by effecting a better adaptation of the worker to his job. Institutions, organizations, and publications of various sorts came into existence for the purpose of forwarding this idea.[1]

The Great Gap in Scientific Management.

The psychological trend in industrial management represented a recognition of the fact that the underlying problem in relating the worker efficiently and satisfactorily to his job could not be solved by an attack upon processes and methods alone. The " law " of diminishing returns had apparently begun to operate. The worker, for a long time looked upon only as a manipulator of materials and a necessary link in a chain of processes, was gradually

[1] Among the organizations which emerged as a part of the scientific management movement the following might be mentioned : (a) The Personnel Research Federation, (b) The American Management Association A.M.A., (c) The Institute of Management, (d) The Taylor Society, (e) The International Management Institute, and (f) The International Industrial Relations Association.

discovered as a physiological organism, and only after this advancement proved insufficient was there a recognition of the worker as a psychic entity.[1] But, important as this move was, it did not reach far enough. It now becomes increasingly obvious that the most significant problems of modern industry lie in the sphere of human relations. Individual psychology aids in an understanding of the relation of the worker to his job, but it omits his relations with other persons. And, the study of individuals, no matter how effectively done, will not furnish adequate information for understanding social problems. Social, as well as individual, psychology is needed.[2]

The great gap, then, in scientific management resides in the fact that it can say nothing about the relations of workers to workers, workers to supervisors, workers to management, management to owners, management to public, et cetera. That is, no scientific data on problems in these spheres now exist. The nature of the problem arising from human relations in industry is not clearly understood. It happens, for example, that in educational institutions one finds departments of industrial research with no psychologists on the staff ; in other institutions courses in industrial relations are attached to departments of economics. These confusions indicate that the real problem of social relationships in industry has not yet

---

[1] The Hawthorne Plant Experiments of the Western Electric Co., *The Personnel Journal*, Vol. VIII, 5, 6 ; Vol. IX, 1.

[2] *Rational Organization and Industrial Relations*, papers by Fledderus and Burns (Publication International Industrial Relations Association), also *The Need for an Applied Psychology of Organization*, H. S. Dennison (Publication of A.M.A., 1925).

been defined. In one sense, it may be true that this clarification awaits more reliable data from the field of social psychology, that no real advance is possible until the social psychologists supply facts and methods which can be put to work on problems as they actually exist in industrial situations.

The Joint Committee epitomizes the Social Problem in Industry.

Employee representation, whatever the motives which brought it into existence in any given industry may have been, constitutes a substitute for the trade union in some of its functions. Where trade unions exist the social problem may be described as a set of relationships between a collective body of workers and a collective body of managers or owners. These relationships are, for the most part, regulated by agreements, or contracts. Actual interaction is confined, ordinarily, to representatives of each collective unit, or group; such interaction, in addition, occurs primarily and almost exclusively during periods of strain or conflict. In industries employing members of organized trade unions provisions are made for bringing social machinery into play when conflict, say a strike, is imminent or in process, but no social mechanisms operate prior to conflict, or in the interest of prevention. Employee representation, its advocates claim, aims to do precisely this, namely, to set in motion permanent and continuing groups whose function is to deal with current problems of relationship, and to anticipate problems likely to precipitate conflict. These continuing groups are joint committees constituted of workers chosen by their fellow-workers and representatives of management chosen by management. These committees become a nexus of relationships between workers and workers, workers and management, and managers and managers. As indicated in the previous chapter, the dualistic structure of these committees, consisting as they do of representatives of two major groups in industry, implies that the principal relationships with which they deal are those between workers and managers.

The joint committee, then, is one of the chief functional aspects of employee representation, and it becomes very important, therefore, to understand the nature and the manner of its operations. Before proceeding in the direction of this understanding, certain reservations and complexities need to be explained. In the first place, it should be clearly understood that these joint committees have been initiated, in most cases, by management and not by workers. Employee representation is viewed by management as an instrument, a tool which management utilizes for the purpose of absorbing and solving the problems of human relationship which arise in industry. In so far as employee representation reveals or goes in the direction of unity, it is a unity the need for which is felt and acted on by management, not by workers. When workers as workers feel the need for unity they organize among themselves but do not include in their membership representatives of employing or managing groups. The joint committee, then, exists because management either needs or believes it needs such social machinery. This fact, while it does not lessen the importance of studying the joint committee's functioning, does condition the entire operation in fundamental ways.

Scientific Management is slow in adopting Psycho-social Research.

Management has been peculiarly reluctant to make use of the tools of psycho-social research. The chief reason for this tardiness is attributable to the nature of the problem itself. Industry passed from small-sized, personally owned and directed enterprises to large-sized, corporate forms very quickly, indeed, so quickly that many industrial leaders still speak of the problem of human relations as though it had not changed at all. Obviously, new approaches to the understanding of the problem cannot be made until there comes into being an objective realization of the altered nature of the problem. So long as management leaders continue to believe that the problem of human relations in industry is exactly what it has always been, namely the adjustment of one individual to another, there can be very little advance.

In the second place, human relations are exceedingly abstract in certain respects; what is involved in these relations is not easily recognized except by consequences, and there are as yet no adequate tests for measuring consequences. Those involved in such relationships do not willingly admit that bad end-results are traceable to their own conduct; they usually fix responsibility elsewhere. Management representatives are themselves involved in joint committees and they find it difficult, therefore, to be wholly objective about their social conduct.

Further, many management representatives and leaders still look upon employee representation in sentimental terms, and it is always difficult to mix science with sentiment. Those who maintain this sentimental attitude are likely to believe that good-will, friendliness, and qualities of this sort will suffice to furnish the proper lubricant for their committees, and this attitude, of course, leads them away from scientific considerations, and especially from seeing themselves as part of the problem. Thus the problems of the joint committee lie very near the total assortment of administrative problems, most of which have thus far escaped scientific scrutiny. These and numerous other factors within the situation of human relationships in industry suffice to explain why the scientific approach has been lacking.[1] But, there is still another reason, and this idea lies on the obverse side of the equation.

Psycho-social Research has its own Confusions.

The nature of human relations in industry is not readily defined, and this because the tools of psychology and sociology—the involved sciences—are still inadequate. The present study is directed toward an analysis of one feature of these relations, namely the joint committee, but even this restricted phase of group process in industry must be approached as hypothesis. It must be candidly admitted that no tested method for studying groups, with respect to their functions, now exists.

[1] *Scientific Management in American Industry*, The Taylor Society, Chapters IV, VIII.

C

Confusion of a very disturbing sort inheres in the fact that social scientists have not as yet decided whether their methods are to be the same or different than those of the physical and biological sciences. Two schools of thought claim the right of way : (a) those social scientists who contend that social phenomena are precisely the same as all other natural phenomena and that consequently social research differs in no way from all scientific research, and (b) those who insist that social relationships involve qualities absent in other natural phenomena and that therefore research methods must be adapted to this distinction. The first group may be called " quantitativists " and the second " qualitativists." This is not the place to elaborate the dispute between these protagonists, but it should be stated that the study which is here presented belongs primarily in the latter classification ; its premises do not deny the ultimate possibility of a social science based wholly upon naturalistic methods, but they do imply that no study of this sort is now possible. In other words, this study proceeds upon the basis that social scientists must first have more authentic knowledge about what it is they are observing before quantitative methods may be validly employed. Certainly, the objective reality of social relationships is still to be unravelled. The time may arrive when all aspects of these subtle relationships may be described in terms of neuronic functions, sugar-content in the blood-stream, glandular precipitates, et cetera, but there are sufficient reasons for believing that even these quantitative measurements will not satisfactorily describe what sort of event is transpiring when human beings interact with each other.

Research in that area of phenomena which can now only be called psycho-social, must operate on the basis of hypotheses. These hypotheses are related both to methods and to the nature of the facts with which they deal.

PART II

DEVELOPING A SOCIAL PHILOSOPHY

HYPOTHESIS OF SOCIAL DYNAMICS

III. IMPULSION

IV. CIRCUMJACENCE

V. INTERACTION

VI. EMERGENCE

PART TWO

EVOLVING A SOCIAL PHILOSOPHY

MUCH of the difficulty in scientific reasoning is to be attributed to the fact that thinkers, especially original thinkers, are likely to regard their categories as absolutes and ultimates. Once they have hit upon a term or phrase which is pregnant with meaning they somehow or other allow their emotions to become attached to the word; they become protagonists for verbal symbols. Words are, of course, nothing but symbols, and concepts are merely tools to be used in reasoning and in communicating meanings to others. The procedure for deriving suitable categories for any given scientific context belongs primarily to philosophy. A " good " category is one which stands meaningfully by itself and at the same time bears an " organic " relation to the whole, that is, the whole of any given set of concepts belonging to a selected area of discourse. Sociologists have experimented with many categories and each generation appears to attach itself to one or more which thereafter become " popularized." The terms which we describe in the succeeding four chapters are to be regarded merely as tools of analysis suitable for the purposes of this study; they carry no other meaning and we are fully aware of their deficiencies even for our aims.

CHAPTER III

THE FIRST ANALYTICAL CATEGORY : IMPULSION

" Empirically speaking, the most obvious difference between living and non-living things is that the activities of the former are characterized by needs, by efforts which are active demands to satisfy needs, and by satisfactions. In making this statement, the terms need, effort and satisfaction are primarily employed in a biological sense. By need is meant a condition of tensional distribution of energies such that the body is in a condition of uneasy or unstable equilibrium. By demand of effort is meant the fact that this state is manifested in movements which modify environing bodies in ways which react upon the body, so that the characteristic pattern of active equilibrium is restored. By satisfaction is meant this recovery of equilibrium pattern, consequent upon the changes of environment due to interactions with the active demands of the organism." —JOHN DEWEY.

GROUPS exist as social forms; human energy has either been appropriated or redirected in order to bring groups into existence. Absence of social forms might be interpreted as social inertia ; likewise decadence of social forms. But since human life does not appear to exist anywhere without the tendency toward social forms, this point does not call for emphasis. Social inertia is not to be interpreted as absence of human energy but rather lack of purpose or skill. Inertia is, consequently, a faulty term as here used since it is made to cover energy displaying itself in random, undirected movements. New social forms arise whenever potential human energy is transposed into kinetic energy as response to a social motive. (If it may be argued that all motives are at

39

bottom individual and that socialization is merely a response to self-interest, this does not alter the equation ; the new social form can only arise when more than one individual is pressed by the same need, and in this sense the motive becomes social.) This redirection of human energy into social channels represents the thrust, the impulse, the dynamics of the social process. By contrast, all tendency toward disability, ineptitude, and quiescence may be thought of as aspects of social inertia. What, then, is the source of this potential human energy which becomes kinetic as it is caught up in social patterns ? This phenomenon of redirection of energy represents the dynamics of social process. By contrast, all tendency toward disability, ineptitude, quiescence may be thought of as social inertia. Our initial query then becomes : What is the source of human energy ? Or, more particularly in terms of our present preoccupation, what is the source of that energy which becomes social dynamics ?

Needs, Wants, Desires and Purposes ; the Basic Factors in Social Dynamics.

The essence of living is function. One need not go beyond this simple statement to find explanations for the fact that organisms have needs, wants, and desires which impel them toward action, and which ultimately get themselves organized as purposes, or interests. An organism can never be wholly quiescent. Activity is always present.[1] Beginning at the bottom, activity is a

---

[1] "Since all of the autonomic apparatus is more or less active all the time, the stream of cravings flowing from its tensions is more or less active ; that is, all of our wishing functions, whether we are conscious

means for satisfying cravings, hungers. But there is a second principle of the organism, namely, the tendency to seek an optimum of functioning. The healthy organism does not stop with the satisfaction of elemental hungers ; it explores and experiments; it often uses prodigious energy in activity which serves no utilitarian end, that is, in play. Consequently, new wants are always on the horizon ; when one level of want has been satisfied, and potential energy is still present, a new level of want will automatically come into existence. This is particularly true of human organisms with highly developed nervous or projicient systems capable of intellectualizing and envisaging new satisfactions.

Human Needs as the Basis of Social Forms in Industry.

Returning now to our task of formulating an hypothesis for the purpose of analysing joint committees in industry, we may begin by stating that no necessity appears for explaining in detail the manner in which individual needs flow toward social forms. There is no mystery in this process ; social forms are merely mechanisms designed to satisfy individual needs. Social organization secures certain satisfactions, makes room for the emergence of

of them or not, are more or less active all the time. *Each moment's behaviour is the resultant of the manner in which the cravings, reinforcing or inhibiting one another, converge upon the striped muscles : hence, upon the sequence of acts or stream of activity, and the content of consciousness."* Psychopathology, by Edward J. Kempf, p. 52.

See also Chapter III, " The Motive of Life is to Function," in *The Science of Social Relations*, by Hornell Hart.

new needs, and consequently becomes an instrument for enlarging and enhancing individual satisfactions.[1]

The trade union is a social form in industry which may be explained in terms of needs, wants, desires, and purposes articulated by workers. The joint committee, as the objective functioning element in employee representation, is partially derived from the trade union : it is designed to allow for the expression of needs, wants, and desires within a collective pattern. There is, however, a difference ; the trade union expresses the needs and wants of its members through demands which may or may not be considered negotiable by management ; in the joint committee all problems are supposed to arise within a conference setting, *i.e.* consistent with and adjustable within the local industrial group. The committee form of organization is, no doubt, partially derived from traditional Anglo-Saxon patterns of social organization. But this is perhaps a minor discrimination. The significant aspect of the joint committee is that it derives the major portion of its dynamic from the needs of the employing or managing group in industry. (The dynamics of workers' needs is, of course, felt indirectly in the joint committee, as will be shown later : one of the aims of management in initiating plans for employee representation, as was

---

[1] Rigid definitions would, probably, be confusing at this point. Tentatively, it may be said that the authors are using these terms, descriptive of the impulsive aspect of conduct, in the following manner : (a) *Needs* are conceived as physiologically derived cravings or hungers ; (b) *Wants* as consciously expressed or elaborated needs ; (c) *Desires* as wants at the point of striving, that is, activated wishes. *Purpose* is a consciously formulated scheme of any or all of the above in terms of goal or end-result. These are, obviously, rough and approximate, as well as arbitrary, definitions.

indicated above, Chapter I, was to canalize the workers' needs in order to prevent its capitalization and manipulation by " outside agitators.")

Traditionally, industrial relations have been thought of as equations with management on one side and employees on the other. The organization of management in modern industry is based upon this conception. Labour organization, trade unionism, is a response to this separation ; trade unions did not originate as stimulus in industry, but rather as response to management's conception of division of function and consequent control. Why, then, do we find in modern industry the trend toward collective forms in which management's needs are prominently displayed ?

From the standpoint of those concerned with industrial relations, management may be said to function under the pressure of three dominant needs, namely (a) a working force adequate in quality, quantity, and stability ; (b) protection from external controls which are antagonistic to the given economic system within which the industry has its legal setting ; and (c) a sustained co-ordination of managerial aims and activities. These needs are, of course, subsidiary to the general need for efficiency and economy in a society, that is, which depends upon private initiative. Given these needs, it seems obvious that management cannot achieve its purposes without securing collaboration from workers.[1] We shall show later how

---

[1] It should be noted here that the principal incidence of employee representation plans came during the period of the War of 1914–18. Indeed, the compulsions of the War Labour Board and the War Industries Board made some form of collaboration between workers and management mandatory. The main need at this time was, of course, stability of the working force.

these management needs intrude themselves upon the operation of joint committees.

The needs of management coalesce readily into a generalized purpose, namely, that of conducting the affairs of an industry with such efficiency as to insure a margin of profit above cost of production. Do the workers have a correspondingly clear and objective purpose ? It is probable that, in the bulk of American industry, no such general purpose exists. Workers, of course, desire to secure for themselves as large a share as possible of the net income from industry, but aside from this highly variable purpose, their major needs remain specialized.[1] In some employee representation plans provisions are made for caucusing among the employee representatives prior to the joint session ; at these caucuses the workers decide upon the wants and desires which they later put before the joint group. This scheme allows for the development of employee purposes, but observation indicates that the problems presented by employees remain, for the most part, indicative of individual and special need. Indeed, many items covering employee wants and desires are introduced by management representatives.

Impulsion as the First Category of Analysis.

All of the above interpretations, designed to explain why joint committees exist, how they come to be the channels of energy, may now be subsumed for reasons of

---

[1] The American Federation of Labour from time to time attempts to formulate the general purposes of the workers but its adherents constitute only a fraction of the total working force of the nation.

convenience under one category. We select for this use
the term *Impulsion*. And, also for reasons of convenience,
we define this category in the following manner :

Impulsion : As a psycho-sociological category, impulsion may be taken to denote all of those aspects of
a group (a social form) which combine to constitute its
initial and ongoing dynamic. The principal analytical
terms of which impulsion is inclusive are needs, wants,
desires, and purposes generated by individual human
beings but expressing themselves in social, or collective
modes.

Any category of analysis should, presumably, be judged
by its capacity to reveal pertinent and relevant facts when
utilized as an hypothesis of observation. In addition, it
should possess the quality of inclusiveness, should be
usable for a wide number of similar phenomena. Besides,
it should not be susceptible of too much ambiguity.
Impulsion appears to be such a term, and hereafter will
be employed to denote the dynamic aspects of joint
committees.

Wherever there is social impulsion there is also the
possibility, if not the likelihood, of *repulsion*. Energy
does not get itself released in a vacuum. Action implies
reaction. It is therefore important to add that schemes
for employee representation, that is, the representation of
employees upon joint committees with representatives of
management, have not been projected without opposition.
Organized trade unions, for example, regard employee
representation as one of the most formidable enemies.
In trade union parlance, employee representation plans

are called " company unions," a term carrying opprobrium, implying as it does that the workers are allowing themselves to be organized in terms of the " company's," not the workers' initiative.   Trade unionists believe that organizations of workers within a single company and not according to crafts or industries as a whole might in the end enslave workers completely ; certainly, many union leaders believe that employee representation is designed mainly as a weapon for fighting organized workers.   Many, if not most, so-called liberals hold this same conviction.   As a result, there has existed a persistent campaign directed against employee representation.

A more subtle form of repulsion operates within employee representation schemes themselves.   The main causes of reaction here are : (a) management's artificial and limited conception of employee needs ; (b) the method used when a joint committee is in session ; (c) over-dominant purposes of management.   Most of these factors of repulsion blend subtly into the total environment in which employee representation plans are obliged to make their way, and this consideration leads in the direction of our next category of analysis.

CHAPTER IV

CIRCUMJACENCE

" . . . the environment if properly analysed is more decisive in determining growth than was formerly conceived possible. The biophysicist need not, therefore, look upon the organism exclusively as a self-controlling and self-perpetuating machine. He can view it also as a reaction-system, *i.e.* a set of reactions between one part of the world and the rest. . . . If we think of growth not as mere unfolding of what is already preformed but as a process of modification through the interaction of the organism and the environment, the original relative simplicity is not an insuperable objection to subsequent complexity."
—MORRIS R. COHEN.

" . . . behaviour in the ordinary sense of the organism as a whole, represents in each particular case a behaviour pattern potentially present in the organism, but realized only through the action of an external factor. . . . Biologically speaking, social integration represents for the individual a reaction to a particular factor in his environment, viz., another individual or group of individuals. We must search, therefore, for the foundations of social integration in the relations of the individual to his environment and more particularly his living environment."
—CHARLES M. CHILD.

Social Forms and the Social Environment.

SOCIAL forms, like the individuals whose needs they express, must of necessity operate within a larger social *milieu.* This *milieu*, conceived as a definite factor of control, like all environment, has its specific elements by which this control is made operative. For present purposes, then, we need a category which will be useful in describing the channels in which our isolated joint committees in industry make their way. Our aim is to describe briefly those selected aspects of the total environment which seem to condition, or limit, or circumscribe, or canalize the dynamics of the joint committee. And, whatever these factors are, we consider them to be interacting elements which modify the functioning of joint committees, and are in turn modified by these committees. Considering the complex interdependence of all factors in the modern world, and particularly with respect to industry, it seems both justifiable and helpful to limit the joint committee's environment to those elements which represent fairly obvious interdependence and relationship.

How Management Philosophy Conditions the Joint Committee.

It was noted above that management purposes, being specific and more clearly defined, exercise a direct and perhaps dominant influence upon the joint committee and its operations. Business enterprise in general is, of course, impossible without purposes of various kinds. These purposes are derived from, or are a part of, a more general outlook on life which characterizes the man who directs business enterprises. Although there is a super-fluity of speculation and opinion with regard to what is " in the mind " of the business man, we have very few authentic facts.[1] Delisle Burns, in his chapter entitled, " The Need for a Psychology of Business Men," [2] writes : " It is possible that the chief psychological fact is their (successful business men) impulse towards realizing their peculiar form of ability in the manipulation of men."

[1] J. D. Houser : *What the Employer Thinks.*
[2] *Industry and Civilization*, p. 269.

If this guess should happen to be true, we should be in possession of a major fact respecting all control aspects of business and industry.

Using a rough classification derived from William James' famous division of the human race, it may be said that there are : (a) "tough-minded," and (b) "tender-minded" managers in industry. When the former dominate in any given concern one discovers that joint committees conform to a rigid mode of operation which, in many respects, is similar to military method. When, on the other hand, the latter type, the sentimentalists in business, are dominant, one witnesses a committee procedure which is almost devoid of conscious methodology ; in these instances, the appeal is not to method, but to goodwill.[1] Where the sentimentalists control, joint committees exist, usually, within a setting of benevolent paternalism ; in the operation of these employee representation plans one frequently encounters the concept of democracy. Where the " tough-minded " (or, in colloquial language, the " hard-boiled ") control, democracy is disavowed ; industry is conceived in terms which disqualify the democratic theory.

Thus it happens that the operation of joint committees in industry is at the outset conditioned by the point of view, the psychology, or the philosophy, of those who are in control. Under the present capitalistically controlled system of industry this is, perhaps, one, if not the most

---

[1] This simple classification into two types of business men is, of course, inadequate. It often happens that a manager who is sentimental with respect to one feature of life is remarkably " hard " with respect to others, and vice versa.

D

important item in the total environment which conditions the joint committee and its functions.

How Employee Psychology Conditions the Joint Committee.

Employees, likewise, bring to the joint committee a variety of attitudes, conceptions, and points of view which materially influence the committee's performance. Many employees, for example, persist in believing that all employers are, to say the least, selfish ; that whatever they propose is designed primarily to advance their interests. They hold this view even toward those employers who appear most benevolent. There are, also, employees of the submissive type who genuinely believe that the employer is always right, that he owns and knows, and is therefore justified in directing without interference.

Briefly, then, our first sub-category of analysis for describing what it is that conditions the joint committee is employer-employee psychologies and philosophies which determine their points of view regarding industrial control and employee-employer relationships.

Committee Structure as Conditioning Factor.

It is commonly believed that social structures are relatively unimportant ; that good results may be attained even with bad structures, providing the proper spirit prevails. Exceptions to this theory need, however, to be made. Structure and functions are interdependent, not separate. A structure is " a definite arrangement and connection of parts with view to a definite function." [1] The very fact that joint committees in industry are constructed according to a dualistic bipartite plan is significant as testifying to the underlying conception of a division of interests which management felt when it designed the particular structure. In certain employee representation schemes provisions are laid down for the actual seating of the delegates—workers on one side and managers on the other. The state of mind which keeps these two groups of representatives divided is in itself a structural fact. Where employees are organized as an " association," and the joint committee becomes only one of the activities of the group, another structural fact emerges. In short, all joint committees exist within a setting of a company structure, an employee representation structure, and a constitutional structure, and this combination of structural facts definitely influences the quality of functioning.

Whenever an employer and an employee consult with each other with respect to a mutual problem, a joint committee may be said to have come into existence. Also, whenever a representative of a trade union, or a group of such representatives, negotiate with an employer, the procedure utilized may be called that of the joint committee. But these are amorphous and often fortuitous committee forms. The joint committee as considered in

---

[1] The structure of the United States Government is embedded in the Constitution ; consequently, numerous difficulties arise with respect to functions ; many of the activities which our Federal Government might engage upon are impossible because of certain structural rigidities, indeed, many of its present functions are the result of a wide liberty in constitutional interpretation.

this study possesses more specific qualities.   A definition
may be useful :

*A joint committee consists of representatives of employees
elected by employees, and representatives of management
chosen by management called into existence as a total
group for the purpose of dealing with certain problems,
usually prescribed in a written constitution.*

Like most definitions, this one is subject to modification.
In some cases, for example, the kind of problems to be
committed to such committees is not specifically prescribed in a written constitution, but is left to the
evolution of experience.   In other cases, no limitations
are placed upon the selection of problems but a very
specific, though informal restriction is practised.   Again,
it will be noted that the above definition implies that
employee representatives are *elected* whereas management
representatives are *chosen*.   The distinction here is borne
out by the facts, but practice is not uniform.

A structural definition should describe " a definite
arrangement and connection of parts, with view to a
definite function," and the above attempt meets these
conditions in a general manner.   It is essential, however,
that this definition should now be given body and content
by way of further and more detailed description.

Structurally, the joint committee conforms to the usual
pattern of a bi-cameral legislative body.   The initial
presumption is this : employees and employers represent
divergent interests, differing points of view, and, perhaps,
a conflicting stake in industry as a whole.   (In this respect
the two groups of representatives are not unlike the

representatives of two dominant political parties in a legislature.) These divergences are, presumably, to be somehow " joined " by the committee process. Management forces in modern industry have come to recognize the need for inner harmony; they are not prepared to concede that the interests of employees and those of management are identical, and consequently, they attempt some form of " balance of powers." The joint committee, therefore, ·is not expected to unify the industry as a whole, but it is expected to reach toward unity with respect to specific issues. In other words, joint committees are to be engaged in the act of unifying without achieving unity.

The precise structural arrangements and connections of various joint committees are not, in themselves, important. In some cases, scrupulous care is taken to provide equal representation, that is, an equal number of employee and management representatives. But this is a naïve conception of representation. Representativeness is qualitative, not quantitative. One management representative with power and authority would be more than equal to twenty employees lacking in power and authority. And, indeed, as will be shown later, management participation in joint discussions is usually confined to one, two, or three persons, and for the most part to the management chairman. Representation among employees invariably follows occupational lines. Each occupational group, department, division, or craft is allotted a specified number of delegates or representatives on a joint committee. In some of the larger industries hierarchies of committees exist and items are referred from " lower " to " higher " committees.

The following diagrams illustrate two of the major types of committee structure found in employee representation schemes :

I.

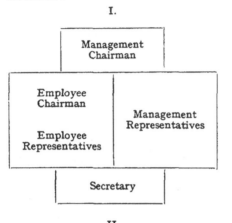

In this type of committee structure, the employee chairman usually functions as presiding officer when employee representatives meet in caucus prior to a joint meeting. The management chairman invariably presides at all joint sessions.

II.

This form is similar to the above with the exception that it provides for dual chairmanship at joint sessions. The employee chairman presides for his group, and the management chairman for his. Certain plans of this type provide that, in case of disagreement, the issue is to be referred to an impartial body.

Facts gathered for the present study, except where noted, relate to committees of Type I. For this reason, a word or two needs to be said regarding the method of operating which prevails when this type of structure is given. Both management and employee representatives, as separate groups, meet previously to a joint session. This pre-conference meeting takes on the form of a caucus ;

representatives, or more often, spokesmen for representatives, are instructed with respect to the attitude which they are expected to assume on questions which it is known will be discussed. Also, they are furnished with items to present before the joint meeting. When the two groups assemble for a joint session a management chairman presides. Discussion then follows until some disposition is made of each item of business. Occasionally, the employee representatives resort to polling among themselves, in which case the employee chairman returns to his rôle as presider for a brief space of time.

It will be noted that this form of joint committee allows for a preponderance of management control and it will be seen later when actual committee process is analysed that the dual position of the chairman is of extreme importance. He possesses at least three major advantages, all of which tend to throw power toward the management side, namely : (a) the prestige which goes with the managerial position ; (b) the inside knowledge regarding management wishes, and (c) the authoritativeness and procedural advantage which accompanies the function of presiding.

Finally, it should be said that a complete understanding of joint-committee structure in any given company should involve an analysis of company structure as well. Joint committees, no doubt, take on something of the pattern of the industry as a whole ; at any rate, company structure obviously reflects itself in joint-committee structure. The present study, however, is chiefly concerned with function, and with structure only in so far as it throws light upon processes.

Conference Procedure as Conditioning Factor.

Most persons who reach the status of managerial responsibility have already formulated a conception of how a committee should be operated. They know " how to run a committee." And, wherever this assurance exists one discovers that the joint committee is by that much limited. If, for example, a management chairman, and most joint committees are presided over by representatives of management, believes that it is his business to see that the committee reaches a conclusion which he has already formulated, many aspects of the problem under consideration will be neglected ; participation will be limited to such comment which suits the chairman's preconceived conclusion, or comment which does not thus conform will be negated. The technique, as well as the validity, of " putting things over " is, then, a fact which must be considered in our evaluation of joint committees.

Some management representatives, conceiving of the joint committee as an opportunity for education, or attitude-changing, will stereotype conference procedure in another way ; those who look upon the joint committee as a means for exchanging experiences, expressing grievances, et cetera, will evolve still another scheme of procedure. In many instances, committee sessions are almost entirely given over to the dissemination of information, and in these cases true conference method, as this procedure is generally interpreted, is not needed. But whatever the conception and the pattern of conference procedure happens to be, it remains as an important conditioner for the committee's functioning.

The Personal Equation Conditions the Group's Functions.

Participants in a joint committee session bring with them certain fairly well-defined habits. These may not be " committee habits " but merely habits of response and stimulus in a social situation. One chairman observed in connection with the present study, for example, had developed the habit of Socratic interrogations ; this habit accompanied him to every meeting, and as chairman he exercised a dominant influence upon the total group. Frequently, committee members are found who habitually respond to all suggestions with negativism ; others have cultivated the habit of acceptance and consequently have lost the habit of criticism. Individual differences are, perhaps, nowhere so important as in social situations where communication proceeds by means of exchange of language symbols, and each difference constitutes a potential limitation to the group's functioning. (The use of the term " potential " in the foregoing sentence is intentional ; if there were no differences there would be no need of committees and conferences.)

The two major individual differences which persons bring to their social relationships are, probably, their intelligence quotient, and what is as yet undefined, their emotional quotient. Nearly all human beings have the same wants and the same sensory needs, but they differ widely in their capacities to express, to strive for, to feel deeply about, that is, to satisfy these needs. In essence, this is what presents us with a social problem, and the committee is a miniature society.[1] The social

[1] See *The Social Basis of Consciousness*, by Trigant Burrow.

problem may be stated as a proposition, namely : Given a wide range of social relativity, a graded series of individual differences, how are we to get on together ? This is essentially the committee's problem.

Psychoses may, or may not be of social origin but in the majority of cases the psychotic person has failed to objectify a social relationship. And psychoses are often found in committees. Because of individual fixations, or blind-spots, or antagonisms, it frequently happens that some member of a committee is wholly incapable of comprehending what another of his colleagues is saying. The " autonomous I " of which Trigant Burrow [1] speaks is conspicuous in committee meetings. It is essentially the unconscious wish to dominate all situations. Interpretation of ideas and therefore understanding of viewpoints and meanings is rendered impossible.

Conclusion : The Second Category of Analysis.

In the previous chapter we considered *impulsion* as a category with which to analyse joint committees, from the point of view of what it is that gives them life. We are now confronted with the necessity of selecting a term which will with some degree of accuracy describe the various conditioning, limiting, channelling factors enumerated above. It will be observed that we are not now dealing with the immediately obvious environment, but particularly with those elements of the conditioning environment which seem to us to be most important as explanation of the joint committee's performance, its

[1] " The Autonomous I in Social Relationships," by Trigant Burrow, *Psyche*, January 1928.

functioning. Five factors have thus been selected, namely: (a) Management attitude and outlook; (b) Employee attitude and outlook; (c) Committee structure; (d) Conference procedure as conception; and (e) The personal equation. These factors do not include a sufficient amount of the total surroundings of joint committees to be called environmental in the sense in which that term is usually employed. Indeed, it is entirely doubtful whether the last-named factor, namely, the personal equation, may be properly considered as environmental at all. The faulty organization of the personalities of conferees, together with their inner " blocks," is certainly an element in impulsion. But we prefer to include certain aspects of the personal equation here because these manifestations of unintegrated personality appear before, and after, and outside the committee setting; they reappear within the committee process as conditioning factors, as phases of the immediate context within which the committee process is obliged to operate. But, it is precisely because of such inconsistencies associated with the term " environment " that we have been led to propose the use of the new category " circumjacence," and we suggest the following definition :

Circumjacence : As a category to be used for psychosocial analysis, circumjacence is the term selected to describe those elements in the total situation which condition, limit, or channel the social group under observation, but only those elements which are reducible to psychological or sociological description.

CHAPTER V

INTERACTION

" The notion of interaction is not simple but very complex. The notion involves not simply the idea of bare collision and rebound, but something much more profound, namely, the internal modifiability of the colliding agents. . . . The situation is not thinkable at all if we do not suppose the internal modifiability of the agents, and this means that these agents are able somehow to receive internally and to react upon impulses which are communicated externally in the form of motion or activity. The simplest form of interaction involves the supposition, therefore, of internal subject-points of their analogues from which impulsions are received and responded to."—ALEXANDER T. ORMOND in *Foundations of Knowledge*.

THE social process, as thus far described, consists of impulsions moving within a given configuration of limiting or circumscribing factors. In a joint committee in industry impulsions derive from the needs, wants, desires, and purposes of participants. If all impulsions arising within the employee as well as the management group were moving in the same general direction, a committee session would consist largely of clarification of needs, understanding of individual differences, and establishing joint means for securing the involved satisfactions. Interaction between participants would, under such conditions, resolve itself into person-to-person relationships, and the quality of such interaction would depend almost wholly upon the degree and significance of individual differences. In the joint committee we are dealing, however, with a

60

more complex form of interaction involving group-to-group as well as person-to-person relationships. Moreover, the two groups cannot be said to be motivated by impulsions going in the same direction. On the contrary, the chief significance of a *joint* committee lies in the fact that impulsions are presumed to be headed toward different, if not opposite, goals. If this were not the case, there might exist a need for committees but not for *joint* committees. We must, then, begin by assuming that interaction within a joint committee is qualitatively different on two levels at least.[1]

Factors in Person-to-Person Interaction.

In one sense it may be said that *the* social problem arises from this fact : each individual human being is different from every other human being ; all individuals are more alike in their needs and wants than in their capacities. Accommodation or adjustment between individuals is difficult in direct proportion to the extent and degree of individual differences.[2] Therefore, unless the individual participants are completely dominated by rule, caucus, or methods of the political machine, individual differences become the primary factors in interaction. A committee session consists of a series of units of communication

[1] Whether or not group-to-group and person-to-person interactions tend to coalesce in joint committees need not be considered here ; hypothetically, we must assume that the two levels of interaction represent two distinct categories. Thus, strictly speaking, there can be no interaction between groups as such. Interaction is always *via* the person, and the *quality* varies as he represents self (person) or other selves (group as in caucus).

[2] For a thoroughgoing treatment of the social significance of individual difference see *Social Psychology*, by Knight Dunlap, Chapters I and II.

between individual persons, and between an individual
and the total group. Each individual communicates in
a mode which is distinct for him; his mode of communication becomes the social stimulus, the initiating
element in interaction. An individual's communicating
mode is always a combination of ideological and emotional
factors which may be represented thus :

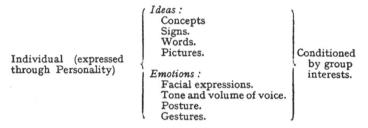

Individual (expressed
through Personality)

Ideas :
   Concepts
   Signs.
   Words.
   Pictures.

Emotions :
   Facial expressions.
   Tone and volume of voice.
   Posture.
   Gestures.

Conditioned
by group
interests.

The formula for interaction may also be presented as
consisting of three kinds of activity expressed by the
interacting personality, namely, sounds, symbols, and
movements. The formula might then appear as follows :

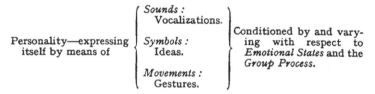

Personality—expressing
itself by means of

Sounds :
   Vocalizations.

Symbols :
   Ideas.

Movements :
   Gestures.

Conditioned by and vary-
ing with respect to
Emotional States and the
Group Process.

For most practical purposes it may be assumed that
interaction within a committee session is to be observed
as a series of stimuli and responses consisting mainly of
ideas expressed in an affirmative or interrogative manner
and conditioned by variables to be found within the
individual personality and the group.

Ideas and emotions are always conjugated, fused and

must be considered jointly as each participant's mode of communication. The quality of interaction is determined, no doubt, by a host of variables all of which go toward making up that entity known as the personality. But whatever this " personality " may be for general psychological purposes, our concern is with the individual as a participant in committee process. Considered specifically, these variants seem to be :

1. The individual's *relation to the problem presented*. If his " stake " in the issue is personal and important, his participation may be expected to be of a distinct quality. Likewise if his relation is one of responsibility as a representative only, or if, for example, he may be involved in the carrying out of the conclusion reached, his participation will vary with respect to the kind of responsibility which he feels.

2. The individual's *knowledge* concerning the item presented. The total group will, obviously, represent zones of knowledge with respect to each given item of business. Other things being equal, it may be expected that participation will be of one kind when knowledge is high, and of another when knowledge is low.

3. The individual's *experience* with respect to this or similar problems. Although it might be assumed that the zone of experience might influence participation directly, the rule does not always follow. In general, however, the quality of participation does vary with experience content.

4. The individual's *emotional set*. This may, of course, be specifically related to the given item, or to a personality involved, or to some factor wholly unrelated to the present discussion.

5. The individual's *attitude pattern*. This may, again, be specific or general. It may be derived from a generalized attitude toward the company as a whole, toward the particular chairman who is presiding, toward the initiator of the item, or toward the utility of committees, et cetera.

6. The individual's *status* as worker, as representative, or as committee member. Those whose status is relatively high do not invariably have a low threshold of response, but their participation, nevertheless, carries a specific quality.

7. The individual's *psychic gradient*. All human relations are, presumably, tinged with pathological potentialities. As sophistication increases, pathological probabilities tend also to increase. Certainly most organized groups, such as committees, are conditioned by psycho-pathologies. Especially to be noted is the tendency toward individual autonomy[1] in which the self remains encased and does not achieve that flexibility of attitude and idea which is needed to raise group process above the superficial into the area of interpenetration.

---

[1] We are indebted to Dr. Trigant Burrow for this concept, as well as for other insights into group process ; his point of view may be reviewed by reference to an essay entitled " The Autonomy of the ' I ' from the Standpoint of Group Analysis," *Psyche*, Vol. VIII, No. 3, January 1928.

The quality of participation for each individual is thus derived from a configuration of these conditioning factors. This may be portrayed in graphic form as follows :

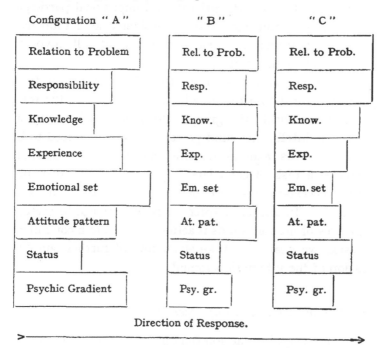

Configuration " A "   " B "   " C "

Relation to Problem	Rel. to Prob.	Rel. to Prob.
Responsibility	Resp.	Resp.
Knowledge	Know.	Know.
Experience	Exp.	Exp.
Emotional set	Em. set	Em. set
Attitude pattern	At. pat.	At. pat.
Status	Status	Status
Psychic Gradient	Psy. gr.	Psy. gr.

Direction of Response.
>————————————————————————————→

While graphic representations are inadequate for purposes of revealing gradations of qualitative responses, the above configurations will, at least, aid in clarifying our meaning. It will be observed that Configuration " B," for example, portrays what might be called " thin " response ; there is no single factor which predominates sufficiently to produce an asymmetrical response. Configuration " A," on the other hand, shows a distinct emotional set ; in this instance the response will be only slightly influenced

E

by the zone of knowledge in which the problem falls for this participant, but emotional bias will be a dominating element. Configuration " C " reveals a response potentially in favour of reasoned, rational, and impersonal participation. The committee process, considered as a total web of participations, is then a blending of all involved individual configurations.

We do not, of course, insist that the above variants as depicted constitute the only factors conditioning the total interaction within the group. Obviously, such factors as sex, age, intelligence, and perhaps racial traits need to be considered as general conditioners, but to disentangle these is a task of considerable proportions and does not seem necessary for our purposes, particularly at this juncture. In a later chapter where we attempt to present the flow of interaction as it actually occurs in a committee session we shall also take steps toward further simplification of the interaction formula.

Factors in Group-to-Group Interaction.

Objectively, interaction can only take place between individual organisms, between persons, or between organisms (persons) and their stimulating environment. If we persist in believing that interaction implies modifiability in both agents, and it is difficult to see how a simple, one-way conception of interaction can be validated, it then becomes logical to include whatever may be regarded as environmental within the equation of interaction. (In Chapter III we have included some of these environing factors under the category of *circumjacence*, but these, and additional factors, are conditioning with respect to interaction as well as impulsion.)

In joint committees each participant responds to and acts upon groups [1] as well as individuals. It is to be noted, for example, that dissension almost never appears within the management group, whereas it frequently characterizes the employee group. Employee representatives, having come to recognize unity in the management group, respond to this unity or solidarity as well as to the individuals constituting the group. There is, then, a *groupness* in a joint committee in terms of which interaction between individuals takes place. Participants for the most part engage in discussions as spokesmen for one or the other group, and often individual desires and ideas are submerged in this interplay of groupness to groupness. In other words, the individuals responding to each other cannot be considered merely as individuals but also as units within a larger social whole. Self-expression in a joint committee is never of the self alone, but always of the self-of-a-group.[2]

---

[1] For purposes of psycho-social research a " group " must be considered as a psychic entity. The use of the term thereby becomes fictional since the collective symbol can only be regarded as a convenience, if not a necessity for individual thinking. It is indispensable as a generalized term. However, it must be kept in mind that the essential reality is the individual's response to this fiction—and not the existence of the entity as such.

[2] Purpose (as clarified expression of the total needs, wants, and desires) must be seen as an important factor in group-to-group response. If, as it sometimes happens, one or both of the groups come into the meeting with a purpose which they do not intend to modify, all the varieties of interaction taking place within that committee must be seen as functions of spoken or unspoken purposes.

The Elements of Interaction.

Adhering to the kinds of joint committees in industry which we have observed, and restricting our hypothesis to this specification for the present, it appears that interaction comprises the following elements :

Individual personalities (as conceived above) who communicate with other personalities by means of ideological signs or symbols, and their emotional concomitants.	This communication varies according to the individual's fluctuating identification with " groups " in which for the time being they find a common purpose or for which they act as representatives receiving ideas and attitudes *en bloc*. This includes the total set of conditioning factors as outlined in the chapters on Impulsion and Circumjacence.

Assuming, then, that primary interaction consists of stimuli and responses passing between individual participants, the equation of interaction may be thus presented :

INDIVIDUAL ◄————————► INDIVIDUAL

His relation to problem ;   His relation to problem ;
His knowledge ;   His knowledge ;
His experience ;   His experience ;
  et cetera.   et cetera.

Group Derivates
Total Impulsion
Circumjacence

The above depicts what happens in an actual committee session : one individual communicates with another in terms of his capacities, his group purpose as involved in the total impulsion, his status as relatively distinguishable

between employees and managers, and in terms of the entire channel (circumjacence) within which committee activities flow. But this picture of interaction does not portray elements sufficiently reduced ; analysis should go at least one step further.

The Analysis of Interaction.

Scientific analysis begins by asking what is the unit to be observed ? What are its properties ? How does it behave ? On first consideration one is apt to be misled by considering the total group, that is, in our case the committee as a whole as the entity for analysis. Any analysis of interaction must be based upon assumptions concerning structure, that is, the properties of the " group " within which it takes place. Physical proximity makes a group in a physical sense only, and since group process or interaction is essentially psychological, the mere aggregation of individuals within a certain space can never constitute a group. Thus, on re-examining the data the hypothesis was formed that analysis must proceed on the basis of the interests represented, and it follows from this that there are as many " groups " as there are interests represented in the total psychic configuration which goes by the name of the joint committee. From this point of view, then, it is apparent that there are generally four major kinds of interest represented :

1. The interest of management as a cohesive group in presenting to the total group some subject related to its purpose.

2. The interest of employees (sometimes as a caucus) who use the joint committee.

3. There are occasional individual interests (which may or may not become items of group importance).

4. There are also common interests upon which the total group can act as a unit.

It appears, then, that since there are as many groups as there are interests, no single set of descriptive categories will be suitable. Thus abstract categories are necessary.

Individual personalities reacting upon each other in a committee session do so in terms of specific situations ; the total group is presented with a problem, confronts a situation, and thereupon engages in discussion. This procedure of communication may be analysed as a series of stimuli and responses. This step brings us nearer categories which are usable in measurement. Total personalities interacting may be used to designate the social process, but for analytical purposes these personalities, plus their impact upon each other, need to be reduced to terms which are more behaviouristic. Our search for such categories has led through a veritable maze of trial and error hypotheses which need not be retraced now.

Interaction, so far as it can be objectively observed, begins with presentation, with oral communication ; the individual who makes the presentation may now be regarded as the agent who releases a social stimulus ; what he is as an individual is still important but only from the point of view of the influence which his personality exercises upon his stimulus. The same is true of response. But, here we confront an added difficulty which renders simple stimulus-response inadequate ; the response which any individual in the group makes to a social stimulus may partake either of that type of reaction known as reflex or of that which is known as reflection. Between these two terms stand many others which represent the total range of varieties of response. In a joint committee, for example, the individual does not respond simply and naïvely as an individual; his response includes some aspects of his rôle as representative, the purposes of his group, his status, et cetera. In short, before he responds overtly, he engages upon a procedure which may be named *organizing his response.* The middle term between stimulus " S " and response " R," namely " O," is peculiarly significant for the social sciences.[1] Stimulus, that is, the manner in which an individual initiates communication with another, may be thought of as being more distinctively a personal and not a social trait. But organization of response may be considered as being primarily a social datum since it is at this point that purely personal ingredients are reinforced by social considerations. When " S " is considered as a constellation rather than as a single stimulus; when " O " is considered as the social mode of organization, and finally, " R " as the total collective response or conclusion to the problem stated in " S," the applicability of the formula S – O – R is evident.

A Final Formula.

As a final formula to be used for purposes of analysis, we have consequently adopted Stimulus-Organization-

[1] For further elaboration of the interaction formula see *The Freudian Wish*, by E. B. Holt, and Chapter XI of *Social Psychology Interpreted*, by J. W. Sprowls; also *Gestalt Psychology*, by Wolfgang Köhler, especially for an interpretation of the middle term, namely, organization of response.

Response, or S – O – R. Each separate item of business transacted by a committee may thus be analysed in terms of its meaning as stimulus, its meaning as organization or social consideration, and finally its meaning as response or conclusion resulting from this organization.

As a category of analysis we may now define *Interaction as that aspect of total social process which includes social stimuli, organizations of response to social stimuli, and overt responses together with the various relations revealed between the three terms.* Since stimuli, organizations of response, and overt responses are not simple forms of interaction, further expression of the formula is necessary. The more precise formula should be $S^n – O – R$, in which S^n indicates a complex stimulus, O the organization preceding response, and R the overt response, and in expanded form this would appear as follows :

$$S^n \; > \!\!-\!\!-\!\!-\!\!-\!\!\longrightarrow \; O \; > \!\!-\!\!-\!\!-\!\!-\!\!\longrightarrow \; R$$

(a) Specific reason or purpose for presenting the item ;	(a) Implicit individual consideration, unspoken ;	(a) Implicit, non-overt, or tacit conclusion ;
(b) The subject-matter represented ;	(b) Explicit individual consideration spoken ;	(b) Explicit, overt conclusion.
(c) The method of introducing the subject ;	(c) Explicit social consideration by means of discussion : (also by means of employee or management caucus.)	
(d) The language mode used ;		
(e) Other aspects of stimulus.		

For a detailed treatment of the content and use of this formula, the reader is referred to Chapter XIV on Statistical Techniques.

CHAPTER VI

EMERGENCE

" What is it that you claim to be emergent ? The reply,
briefly, is : Some new kind of relation."
" Now in order that there shall be a difference in the course
of events the relatedness in question must be what I shall call
effective. By this I mean that when it is present some change
in the existing go of events occurs which would not occur if it
were absent." —C. LLOYD MORGAN.

EQUIPPED with three major categories of analysis, namely,
Impulsion, Circumjacence, and *Interaction,* we are in
position to describe what impels the joint committee in
industry, what canalizes this impulsion as immediate
environment, and what form of movement (action and
reaction) is thereby set going. These are presumed to be
categories suitable for analysing the dynamics of social
phenomena. The consequences of any specific impulsion
operating within a given circumjacence and by means of
a specially conditioned form of interaction need now to
be considered.

The Concept of Social Change.

The term " social change " as popularly used in the
social sciences usually carries one or the other of two
meanings, namely: (a) alterations in culture, or civilization,
compared with some more constant factor, such as man's
biological evolution,[1] or, (b) statistical measurement of
the growth of populations, institutions, social events,

[1] See *Social Change,* by W. F. Ogburn.

73

et cetera.[1] In the first instance change is interpreted in value-terms, its exposition is interfused with judgments. In the second case, changes are merely enumerated. Each science, presumably, must select its own concept of change as well as its own methods of measurement. Ultimately, the aim of all science is to measure change, but this very aim introduces a most subtle element into scientific thought. "There is always something that the human being wants to know," says Ogburn,[2] and it is precisely because he "wants to know" that his emotional prejudices and biases invade his scientific procedures.

What, then, do social scientists wish to know? Obviously, they wish to discover which aspects of social phenomena remain relatively constant and which are relatively flexible, at what rate change takes place, and what causes the change. If the social sciences were to restrict themselves to this list of objectives, they might secure status in the family of the sciences by producing an adequate body of descriptions and statistical analyses. It would then be left to others, moralists and philosophers, perhaps, to discriminate between "good" and "bad" change, between progress and retrogression. We do not believe that social scientists, nor any other scientists for that matter, are capable of restricting themselves in this fashion. The functioning of the human mind is not so simple as this separation implies; we are not able to abstract our judgment from the rest of reasoning at will; nor does our desire for knowledge, that part of us that "wants to know," confine itself wholly to the quantitative.

[1] See *Recent Social Changes*, edited by W. F. Ogburn.
[2] *Ibid.*, p. vi.

It is our contention that what people really want to know is always at some point qualitative and specific ; they desire to know what difference change makes to them and to their lives. Change in time and space is an essential concept and probably underlies all other conceptions of change, but ultimately we all wish to know the meaning of change in relation to our activities and our sense of values.

Change and Emergence.

The term " change " is, perhaps, inadequate for expressing qualitative movement. (Change is, of course, a more general term than movement, since the latter term connotes merely alteration of position in space.)[1] Our specific need is a category which will denote, or at least be inclusive of, the qualitative consequences of interaction. Interaction between non-mechanical entities implies a modifiability on the part of the entities themselves and upon the circumjacent factors. An adequate term for our present purposes would be one which gave meaning to the modifications observable in the interacting participants of joint committees, in their activities as committee members, and in their relation to the groups of which they are functioning parts, namely, the committees themselves. *Emergence* appears to us to be such a term, and we propose to use it hereafter as a category of analysis for purposes of denoting changes in the interacting process as a total situation and as a set of relations.

The search for emergent qualities resulting from social

[1] See *Scientific Thought*, by C. D. Broad, p. 406.

interaction becomes at one stage or another a selective, valuing procedure. Such search will be pointed toward significant change and wherever significance is ascribed valuation has begun. At this point values as resident in the situation and values as inhering in the personality of the research agent converge, but a fuller discussion of this feature of research is reserved for the two succeeding chapters.

Emergence as Related to Previous Categories of Analysis.

Perhaps the most practical method for giving meaning to the term " emergence " as a psycho-social category is to indicate its relation to the three foregoing categories of analysis.

(*a*) Impulsion deals with the energies utilized by joint committees in industry. As a term of analysis, impulsion implies queries concerning the nature of the needs, wants, and desires of both employees and managers ; queries concerning the purpose of each party, and the purposes of both parties considered as a whole.

(*b*) Circumjacence deals with the forms which limit or canalize this energy. Are these forms fixed or flexible ? Are the attitudes and conceptions of management subject to influences exerted by employees, and vice versa ? What variations occur in company organization, employee representation plans, joint committee structure, committee chairmanship, committee procedure, committee habits, et cetera ?

(c) Interaction deals with the quantity and quality of participation in the committee process. Does the quality of participation change ? Do committees advance from simple to complex problems ? Is learning to be observed in the responses made ? Are the more subtle forms of relationship within the group recognized ? Does the flow of interaction lead to changing modes of committee procedure ?

(d) Finally, it must be asked : Does interaction lead to committee decisions which may be qualitatively tested ? It will be seen at this point that a qualitative interpretation of interaction at once leads to the problem of consequences, or emergents. In addition to the quality of committee decisions, one sees at once the necessity of asking such questions as the following : Does the process increase or diminish the separateness of the two collaborating groups, employees and managers ? Is unity or disunity the chief qualitative distinction of emergence ? If unity in anything like a pure sense is not observable, do these joint committees reveal, as a consequence of their interactions, new qualities of relationship ?

Summarizing, then, it appears that changes or emergences may be discovered in impulsion, in circumjacence and in interaction. (Other types of change are present but these three areas appear to be appropriate for a study such as we have conducted.) We may now name these emergents in accordance with their relation to the previous categories, namely, Impulsion-Emergents, Circumjacence-

Emergents, and Interaction-Emergents.   An illustration in each area may suffice to make the meaning clear :

(a) *Impulsion-Emergent :*   A more or less informal joint committee discussion led to the mention of waste in the plant ; this in turn led to a joint investigation of managers and employees of the waste situation and its relation to the welfare of each.   Since this consequence involved needs, wants, and desires, it may be said to have had the effect of altering the impulsion connected with joint committees. In another company the management was so slow in making certain changes requested by the employees that the employees lost interest in the joint committees and meetings lagged.   Here, then, is an illustration of negative impulsion.

(b) *Circumjacence-Emergent :*   In one company a practice has arisen which leads to a periodic revision of the book of rules guiding the work methods of the plant, and it was discovered that this practice arose from discussions in joint committee meetings. The environmental aspects of the total situation were, that is, altered through the activities of joint committee interactions.

(c) *Interaction-Emergent :*   Perhaps the most significant type of emergence is that which may be observed as flowing directly from the interactive process itself.   Under this caption we may distinguish roughly the following types :

(1) Emerging quality of participation ; recognition of personality differences ; level of attention

and interest, problem - solving capacity, et cetera.

(2) Changing recognition of inter-relationships ; employees as a group with managers as a group.

(3) Changing quality of decisions ; increasing or diminishing jointness in the decisions ; level of attention with respect to the " best " as distinguished from the " easiest " solution of a problem.

(4) Changing character of committee procedure ; less or more arbitrary.

(5) Changing character of committee procedure as dominated by the chairman, et cetera.

(6) Changing attitudes toward industrial management; on the part of employees or managers, et cetera.

(7) Changing conceptions of the nature of unity or disunity within industry ; unity as possible, or unity as becoming but never arriving, et cetera.

An illustration of at least one of the above emergents may be found in the fact that many management officials and technologists interested in industrial management are now directing their attention to the problem of committee procedure ; this concern has grown directly from considerations involving joint committees. Since this current interest comes directly within the scope of the present study, we may include further comment. There are, it appears, three schools of thought among industrialists with respect to committee procedure ; and these may be designated in the following manner :

(a) Those who adhere to a modified *Socratic Method*.

Through the use of this type of committee procedure the chairman trains himself in question-
asking ; he seldom makes affirmative statements
but gradually reveals the attitudes, opinions, and
experiences of the members of the group by means
of advancing interrogations. Under guidance of
this sort from the chairman agreement usually
arrives as common assent.

(b) Those who adhere to the so-called *Developmental
Method*. This type of committee procedure is, no
doubt, an outgrowth of Socratic techniques. It
operates as development of any given problem
by a mixture of questions and affirmations put
by the chairman. He decides in advance what
the proper solution to the problem is, and then
guides the group by skilful manœuvres to this
conclusion.

(c) Those who adhere to the so-called *Discussion Method*.
This newer type of committee procedure should,
perhaps, be called the " educational method,"
since it is based upon a pedagogical principle,
namely, the notion that interest in a learning
experience can only be maintained at a fruitful
level when the participants are dealing with a
true problem and when they approach it in the
mood of discovery. This principle of so-called
" progressive education " includes far-reaching
corollaries of both a philosophical and a methodological character. The use of discussion as the
instrument for actually discovering solutions in

committees implies a kind of faith in human nature which is absent in the two above methods ; the chairman becomes the teacher who guides the procedure but not with respect to the end, or solution ; he stands prepared to abide by the consequences of the conclusion which represents the group, its knowledge and its purpose ; his attention is focused upon method, upon the means which the group utilizes in reaching its decisions.

This is not the place, obviously, to discuss fully these various schools of thought, each of which has its devotees in industry. Very few joint committees utilize the last-named method. Discussion is still regarded as a procedure of questions and answers in which the chairman does the answering.[1] The Developmental Method, on the other hand, is widely used in joint committees and many chairmen have reached a high degree of skill in its application. The reader will have become aware that the kinds of consequences, emergents, which may be expected from a joint committee are in large measure dependent upon the type of procedure utilized in the committee's deliberations.

Are Committee Emergences Measurable ?

The committee as an instrument of social control is of such importance that it seems necessary to approach the task of measuring its consequences. Certainly, industrial leaders will sooner or later be brought to this realization

---

[1] For elaborations of the Discussion Method, see *Training for Group Experience, Creative Discussion,* and other Inquiry publications ; see all *The Technique of Group Discussion,* by Harrison Elliott.

F

by reasons of economy. The discussion of committee emergents is futile unless accompanied by further consideration of how these end-results may be reduced to terms of comparability. In the present study considerable time and effort was directed toward this problem, and although we are not prepared to make specific proposals we shall include several suggestions which may prove useful to other investigators and experimenters.

No universal measurement for committee output is now available, nor are we able to propose one. Our measurement experiments have merely been carried to the point where it seems feasible to compare committees within the same company. Our S–O–R formula for analysing the dynamics of committee process may be universally used but something needs to be added to make emergents comparable as between different industrial units. This situation arises because of the divergences in underlying philosophies of industrial management ; each company acts in relation to a given, and in most instances a traditionally derived, conception of control ; consequently, each company expects varying degrees of participation from its managers, technologists, and workers. This quality of expectation reaches all the way down to joint committees and modifies both the procedures for each committee in each separate company and also the emergent potentialities.

Within a given company, however, standards of various sorts may be arbitrarily agreed upon and committees of all grades may be tested with respect to their output as measured by such standards. Agreement may be reached, for example, with respect to what constitutes higher and lower types of problems ; each type of problem coming before a committee would then be weighted and a committee would be rated according to the amount of its time spent upon problems presumed to have greater or lesser importance to this particular industry. A tentative classification of this sort is placed in the footnote below.[1]

[1] The various items of business conducted by a joint committee may be classified as follows :

(1) *Gratuitous, Expository Fact.*—Consisting of expressions of an individual directed to the group but without attention to the group's interests ; there is no response, the committee members act as listeners to information which is unsolicited. (This type of item occurs usually at the beginning or near the close of session, or when no active discussion is under way.)

(2) *Routine Committee Procedure.*—Consisting of the reading of minutes of preceding meetings, reference to previously considered items, or announcements ; interest centres primarily about the accuracy of the record, but overt response is not usually forthcoming.

(3) *Focused Conversation.*—Unpremeditated interaction, but focused upon a single subject ; this may consist merely of questions and answers, no important problem is under consideration, and the procedure is informal.

(4) *Requested Information.*—Consisting of actual and formal committee business initiated in the form of a question asked by one person ; the answers may be furnished by one or more participants ; attention is directed to a single problem and interests of participants are revealed.

(5) *Sympathetics.*—Consisting of either diffuse or specific expressions of sympathy by the group on behalf of some person or persons ; expressions of goodwill, gratitude, condolence, or commendation usually presented without much consideration and involving no elements of conflict.

(6) *Anticipatory Information.*—Information furnished (usually by a management representative) in anticipation of a latent misgiving or conflict ; this type of information often leads to the discussion of a real problem, but the implication is that the situation involved may be clarified by an understanding of facts.

(7) *Direct Requests.*—Consisting of requests (made usually by employees) concerning things, services, conveniences, et cetera ; the expected conclusion is forecast in the statement of the request.

(8) *Explicit Complaints.*—Expressed dissatisfactions but not necessarily implying or forecasting the solution ; the committee is utilized,

Another scale of measurement might be based upon an arbitrary set of values ascribed in advance to the quality of decision reached by the committee with respect to true problems, that is, problems for which the committee is expected to find solutions and for which it exercises acknowledged responsibility.   But, what values may be appropriately utilized for such a purpose ?   Some have proposed and indeed studies have been premised upon a single value, namely Democracy.   This is, of course, a blanket term and may indicate a variety of meanings ; usually, however, the term " Democracy " serves as a rough test of the committee's procedure.   If the workers are actually allowed to participate candidly, if their opinions are taken into account, and if in the end the solution arrived at by the committee belongs as much to

when confronted with items of this sort, for purposes of finding or of sanctioning a solution.

(9) *Proposals.*—Consisting of propositions laid before the committee in which probable solutions have been devised in advance ; proposals do not ordinarily grow out of current requests or complaints but come in anticipation of desired action ; a specific solution is not always expected but the committee is given the task of developing the underlying and relevant ideas.

(10) *Policy-making, Problems.*—Consisting of negotiations designed to lay the basis for future relationships ; this type of item may grow out of 4, 5, 6, 7, and 8, or may be initiated as the search for a principle when no specific situation is involved.

Examination of the above items indicates that Numbers 1 to 6, inclusive, are of one general type, whereas Numbers 7 to 10 represent another. In ordinary committee procedure items of the kind described under categories 1 to 6 do not evoke discussion because they are not indicative of conflict or difference ; these are the types of items which occur in committees simply because there exists a delegate body, primarily as a matter of routine.   Obviously, the consummations, or emergent results derived from the introduction of such items are not of the same importance as those implicit in items of the types described in Numbers 7 to 10.

employees as to managers, all of this is regarded as a democratic procedure. The test is also applied to methods of electing employee representatives, the degree of freedom granted employees in making complaints, et cetera. But, it seems to us that Democracy is much too ambiguous a term to be used as a part of research. Its overtones and undertones call forth too many notions which are embedded in emotional biases.

Underneath the term "Democracy," and probably as a more refined conception, may be found a wider range of values which describe more accurately the qualitative possibilities of social action. For example, where one person stands to another in the relation of subordinate, the process of interaction according to which they arrive at conclusions may consist of commands and obediences. So far as external observation goes, this form of interaction represents a one-way process ; the subordinate person exercises no influence upon the decision, and his personality, his desires, wishes, interests, purposes, are not taken into consideration. The person in authority, in cases of this type, directs an external stimulus toward the subordinate, and he expects the subordinate to *acquiesce*. If, stepping to a slightly higher plane, the person in authority makes his suggested decision in the presence of the subordinate and at the same time allows for comment, the resultant conclusion may be termed *assent*. The former quality, acquiescence, is usually found in military organizations and in the relations between parents and young children. In the case of children it invariably happens that growth itself, that is, the evolution of the child's personality, makes it necessary for parents to step from acquiescence to assent. When real differences begin to appear in social relationships, differences founded upon divergent interests, it usually appears that one side or the other is prepared to accept less than it demanded at the outset, providing the other side is in turn prepared to make a similar sacrifice. This type of conclusion may be called a *compromise*. Before a compromise may be reached, a two-way process of interaction must have transpired, differences must have been at least partially explored, and it must have been assumed that authority to decide was in some measure joint and not vested wholly in one or the other of the engaged parties. When the same two-way process of interaction culminates in a conclusion in which no sacrifices have been made, in which both groups have attained what they really wanted, the result may be called *consent*. And, when the consenting mode is carried so far as to lead the participants to invent a new conclusion not hitherto proposed by separate individuals, the result may be called *integration*.

The above terms furnish us with a graded system of values, and although considerable subjectivity clings to these concepts, they may be utilized with more accuracy than a blanket term such as " Democracy." To ask if a social form or a social process is democratic is too much like asking an individual if he is good or bad. And, perhaps, this is the place to state that we are not here proposing an ultimate scheme of values. Indeed, it is not congenial to our way of thinking to assume that values can ever be final and ultimate. The above relativistic values are based upon the assumption that acquiescence, assent, compromise, consent, and integration bear some direct relation to the total configuration of values in contemporary life and culture. We have, in other words, merely added a semi-functional content to a graded system of values which, in a somewhat unrecognized form, already exists. Historically, the American political experiment was designed, partly at least, to allow for *consent*, and perhaps in no other country of the modern world is there so much theoretical discussion of the means for eliminating arbitrary authority. We are not blind to the fact that in actual practice arbitrary authorities may be found in abundance ; but a value always partakes somewhat of an ideal, representing as it does a judgment between the less-good and the better. But, in so far as we apply these criteria of value to items dealt with by joint committees in industry we presume merely to indicate a trend, a gradient ; we do not presume to state that every item presented to a committee is susceptible of, let us say, an integrative conclusion.

A Proposal for Discovering Emergence.

Granted that the above set of values as attached to the concluding stage of committee process is valid for its cultural setting, how may it be utilized for purposes of testing emergence ? These imputed values are, of course, pertinent only for committee items representing actual or potential adjustment between individuals, between departments, between employees and management, et cetera. Obviously, the first correlation to be made is that between the kind of situation and the quality of conclusion. Do committees find it possible to deal more creatively with certain items than others ? In the

second place, the quality of conclusions reached by any
given committee must be referred to the background of
employee representation in the company ; some management groups, for example, specifically disavow any
intention to develop inventiveness and creativeness
through committees. And, in the third place, the qualities
of conclusions must be related in each instance to the
specified function of the particular committee in question ;
if, for example, the committee is instructed to serve only
in an advisory capacity, its decisions will not be the same
as they might be if the committee were actually instructed
to legislate. In view of the above variables, our scheme
of values becomes still more relativistic, but we present
it, nevertheless, as hypothesis. The diagram below may
serve to further clarify this conception of graded values as
attached to committee conclusions :

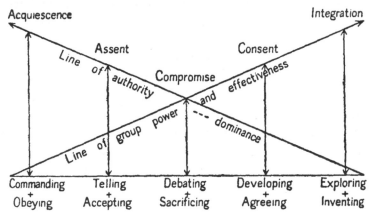

The above diagram indicates three aspects of committee
process, each representing a phase of quality, or value ;
the two heavy diagonal lines, one going to the left and the

other to the right, indicate, respectively, direction toward arbitrary authority and toward group effectiveness; the horizontal lines pointing upward indicate types of conclusions possible arranged in a graded scale reaching from acquiescence to integration; and pointing downward, these same lines indicate the kind of activity which engages the committee when it arrives at each type of conclusion.

All decisions reached by a joint committee are important, provided they emerge as action. In Chapter II we insisted that the only objective point of view from which joint committees might be considered was that of their rôle as instruments of management. Therefore, a precise measurement of the results of committee action would trace these beyond the committee session to discover how they finally emanated as action. If, for example, a management representative submits to the employee representatives a series of possible solutions for a situation, and asks them to discuss these in the light of relative choices, the advice which he secures may be a very small part of the actual conclusion, but it, nevertheless, gets itself incorporated in action, and is, therefore, significant. In the diagram below it will be seen how even advisory functions of joint committees become a part of the total management in industry:

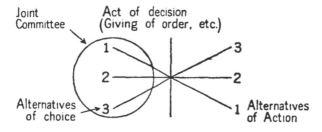

Still another proposal for analysing the output of joint committees might be devised by establishing correlated weightings, that is, by bringing each type of subject-matter or committee business confronted by the committee as a true problem into relation with the above value scale. If, for example, the higher types of conclusion are reached only with respect to the less-valued types of problems, the committee would be regarded as functioning at a low level of efficiency, and vice versa.

As a category of analysis we may define emergence in the following language :

Emergence represents any evolutionary change in the quality of the consequences of joint committee action observable in the committee's impulsion, circumjacence, and interaction.

PART III

CLARIFYING SOCIAL METHODOLOGY

PART THREE

CLARIFYING SOCIAL METHODOLOGY

THE path from philosophy to scientific method is filled with hazards. Most thinkers prefer to travel in the opposite direction ; they place their feet firmly on the assumed facts of science and construct therefrom whatever general principles and philosophical concepts appear as warranted. But, to see one's philosophy as involved in, and not separate from, as precedent to one's science, reverses the procedure and multiplies the difficulties. Now and then such a reversal becomes an essential part of thought, both for the individual and for the thinkers of a given period of time. It represents a sort of intellectual renovation, and at the same time allows one to bring the two essential strands of thought into a relationship of renewed harmony.

The transition from philosophy to science involves at least two stages, namely, a clarification of the problem of epistemology and a rationalization of the place of the observer, the percipient, in the fact-finding process. It was thought for a time that the so-called " New Realists " had somehow settled the epistemological problem in so far as scientific thought was concerned ; we now see, however, that their pronouncements were both premature and over-affirmative. And this is encouraging, since it may aid us to see also the fallacy in hoping for final solutions of philosophical problems ; there are no such solutions, and each age of cultural distinction must find signposts of its own. And on all sides we begin to note the indications of disintegration of the naïve philosophy of an independent fact-finder standing somehow pure and purposeless aside from the facts with which he deals. Hence the philosophical task confronting scientists becomes pertinent and imperative.

CHAPTER VII

VALUES AND SUBJECTIVITY IN SOCIAL RESEARCH

(*An Epistemological Note*)

" A crude fact is not scientific."   —CLAUDE BERNARD.

" If the student means to try the experiment of framing a dynamic law, he must assign values. . . ." —HENRY ADAMS.

" Similarly, and in a more general way, we cannot conceive of a scientific fact without an observer to express it. Equations do not exist in nature any more than colours or sounds. There is something, unknown to ourselves, which our ears translate into sound, our eyes into colour, our mind into equations. Had our rational ego been different, the scientific image of the world would have been different, just as visual images for the colour-blind are."   —JACQUES RUEFF.

THE foregoing categories—*Impulsion, Circumjacence, Interaction,* and *Emergence*—are representative of social hypothesis. These are the postulates which we propose to utilize as symbols for the dynamics of social process.

Our problem by way of recapitulation is the joint committee in industry ; our aim is to describe the functioning, the dynamics, of these committees ; our hypothesis may be said to consist of the notion that dynamics proceeds from some source, is the result of social factors, which we call *Impulsion* ; but social forces do not operate in a vacuum ; they are circumscribed and conditioned by various environments, several of which we have selected for our purposes and named *Circumjacence* ; social impulsions as conditioned by their environments reveal themselves in the form of stimuli and responses,

93

actions and reactions, between human beings ; these we have called *Interactions* ; interactions, in turn, produce certain changes all along the line, changes in the interaction process itself, changes in circumjacence, and in impulsion ; these emanating changes we have named *Emergences.* How may these categories of hypothesis be utilized as categories of methodology ?

A sound hypothesis will give forth trustworthy facts only when put into use through a valid method. But what constitutes valid method for the social sciences ? Although it may appear as tautology, a valid method for any science is one which reveals valid knowledge with respect to the appropriate problems of that science. This more or less obvious statement does not, however, completely clarify our situation. What is needed is a clearer notion of the concept of *validity*, and this carries us directly into the area of epistemology.

Josiah Royce was in the habit of saying that " the epistemological problem . . . is the question as to how we transcend the subjective in our knowledge." The assumption here is that valid knowledge is that from which all subjectivity has been eliminated. But where is such knowledge to be found ? Theoretically, it must be granted that " two hemispheres of reality " exist, namely objective and subjective, but by what empirical process may these be separated ? How does the scientist divorce his thought from his object ? How, indeed, can there be an object for him if he does not perceive (think about) it ? That objects do exist without his thought must be taken for granted, but such existence has no importance, is purely theoretical. The existence of an object becomes important when recognized either as perception or conception. Cognition is the beginning of significance. But cognition is a psychic act; its impulse comes, not from purified reason, but rather from will and wish. " It must be remembered," writes Hans Vaihinger, " that the object of the world of ideas as a whole is not the portrayal of reality—this would be an utterly impossible task—but rather to provide us with an instrument for finding our way about more easily in this world. Subjective processes of thought inhere in the entire structure of cosmic phenomena." [1] The real problem of epistemology, then, is not to find ways of transcending the subjective but rather of including it as a necessary concomitant of what is commonly designated as objective knowledge. Social scientists have not found it easy to accept this point of view. They have, for the most part, attempted to imitate the methods of the physical sciences in which the subjective element appears, superficially at least, to have been conquered. This " wish " for " pure " objectivity [2] still dominates most of what goes by the name of social science. It should not be necessary to recapitulate the complete argument for the subjective-objective view of reality, but enough must be said to make our position clear.[3]

[1] *The Philosophy of As If*, p. 15.

[2] " To know facts solely for the sake of knowing them, out of pure curiosity, is an obsession that haunts Europeans only ; it is this obsession which causes us to suppose a manner of being for phenomena in themselves as phenomena—what we call Objectivity."—Masson-Oursel in *Comparative Philosophy*, p. 190.

[3] For those who may desire to reformulate the argument for themselves we make the following references : (a) *The Philosophy of As If*, by Hans Vaihinger ; (b) *Pragmatism*, by William James ; (c) *The Technique of Controversy*, by B. B. Bogoslovsky ; (d) *The Quest for Certainty*, by John Dewey ; (e) *The Freudian Wish*, by E. Holt ;

In the first place, the social sciences are peculiarly susceptible to subjectivism, and for this reason these disciplines cannot wholly divorce themselves from control-ideas. The term " social " is in and of itself a value-concept ; all efforts directed toward an analysis of what is social, and how the social in existence operates, are either candidly or by implication motivated by the underlying desire for control. And, as Bogoslovsky insists, " as far as we are interested in control, we must be relativists." The wish for control-knowledge inevitably injects a subjective element into social research. (We are here emphasizing the social sciences but, as Hans Vaihinger and Bertrand Russell point out, the same relativism holds true in varying degrees for all the sciences.) The cult of " knowledge for its own sake " is accepted because it feeds a certain human vanity ; based as it is upon a wish, the desire to be accredited with disinterested fact-finding, this search for the purely objective, the non-psychic reality, leads scientists to decorate themselves with false haloes. But the simplest of epistemological exercises quickly reveals the fictional character of this wish. When, for example, a scientist utilizes a word, a term of language, to convey his meaning, he is already engaged in a subjective process. He some-times misleads himself and others by counting these language symbols (statistics), but this in no manner

(f) *Social Discovery*, by E. C. Lindeman ; (g) *The Social Basis of Consciousness*, by Trigant Burrow ; (h) *Meaning of Meaning*, by Ogden and Richards ; (i) *Substance and Function and the Einstein Theory of Relativity*, by Cassirer ; (j) *Emergent Evolution*, by Lloyd Morgan ; (k) *The History of Materialism*, by F. A. Lange ; (l) *Science and the Modern World*, by Whitehead.

relieves him from the obligation of dealing with relative, subjective symbols which cannot convey accurate, precise and constant meanings.

In the second place, the social sciences deal with phenomena of experience. Whatever these sciences may formulate as law or principle must first have passed through an experimental stage. And, all experience is imbued with subjectivism. There is, first of all, *my* experience, about which I cannot possibly be completely objective, impersonal; there is, second, *your* experience, which I can only know at one stage removed; and there is, thirdly, *our* or *their* experience, which is likely to be still another step away from " pure " objectivity. The wish to know this experience which is social is in itself derived from subjective sources, and he who pursues the wish and actually attempts to fathom the nature of social experience must again submit to a subjective procedure; he must, that is, construct certain hypotheses which seem to him to denote what is involved in social phenomena. His hypotheses, in turn, are formulated in terms of relative symbols, concepts, which he arbitrarily employs for purposes of revealing the sort of reality which he has, *a priori*, envisaged. In this study, for example, we have hypothecated the concept " impulsion " which, for us, is a generalization, an abstraction to denote that particular social thrust arising from human needs, desires and purposes responsible for generating employee representation and, in turn, joint committees. Other terms would, no doubt, do as well, but this one seems to suit our purposes and represents as much verbal accuracy as we are capable of utilizing. Our procedure at this stage was, of course,

G

logical, not epistemological. But, even at this point, our logic is relativistic ; we suggest merely that there are probable causes for social phenomena and that these, whatever they are, may be subsumed under a single category provided it is sufficiently abstract, generalized.

If the social sciences were capable of employing a purely objective method of research, all that would be needed for purposes of validity would be de-subjectivized, de-personalized " spectators " who could dispassionately observe events, analyse their various aspects, and reduce their findings to statistical forms. But it is precisely this " spectator " knowledge [1] which is to be mistrusted. The " scientist " who is capable of so much delusion, so much fictionizing, will most certainly allow his unconscious purposes and wishes to intrude. He will, of course, vehemently deny that this is true, but his denial is part of his romantic wish. To admit that his psyche has been involved in his research is tantamount to ruling him out as scientist. The social scientist who utilizes the spectator method becomes a sort of " detective " who spies upon furtive events but keeps himself aloof, free from con-tamination. It is our contention that in so far as his " detective " methods succeed he will, in the same proportion, separate himself from that reality which is significant.

Most of what has been written above may appear to be negative in purport. Because of the persistency with which naïve objectivity continues to influence social research this course seems necessary. If our position regarding subjective-objective research could be made

---

[1] *The Quest for Certainty*, by John Dewey.

clear in a single paragraph, we should be happy to employ such brevity. But, unhappily, the preponderant emphasis in the field of social science is still in the opposite direction. We must, however, proceed to the formulation of our positive argument.

If the subjective element is to be inclusive in social research, the first compulsion of the scientific observer is self-awareness. (Although subjectivism may be attributed to physical, physiological, and psychological spheres, we are here primarily concerned with psychological sub-jectivity.) [1]

Perhaps the most direct way to approach the analysis of the subjective is through an examination of the various kinds of conditionings to which any one individual has been inured throughout his life. That is, his " self-awareness " cannot be a mere getting into the proper mood of repose, there to await those reflections which pour in upon him. But rather it must be dynamic in terms of the wish or purpose of the individual and the kind of value-sets he has acquired. If these conditionings are examined they will be found abstractly to be of two kinds ; first, *personal*, in terms of himself as a psychic entity, why he is in many respects unique as an individual, and how he, as distinguished from others, happened to be what he is. This is largely a matter for determination

[1] " It is then found that subjectivity is of three kinds, physical, physiological, and psychical. The first of these is satisfactorily dealt with by the theory of relativity : the method of tensors is its complete theoretical solution. The second and third are perhaps not really distinct ; they can be dealt with in so far as one man's perceptions differ from another's, but it is difficult to see any method of eliminating subjective elements in which all men are alike "—Bertrand Russell's Int. to Lange : *History of Materialism*, p. xviii.

through the concepts and methods of individual and abnormal psychology.

His conditionings are secondly *social* in terms of the particular *milieu* in which his personal conditionings have been effected. These are what make him behave like, for instance, a European, a Frenchman, a Parisian, as distinguished, say, from an American, an Easterner, a New Yorker. It is these social conditionings which make him a man of his day and time.

For general purposes, a discussion of the conditionings of the individual would end here, but in terms of research we have one other class, namely, scientific conditionings which make him a member of this or that school of thought ; an adept in this or that technique of research.

Thus our conception of self-awareness must always be considered in relation to psycho-social research and the research agent is obliged to ask himself questions such as these :

1. What are the probable factors in my behaviour which make me different from other individuals and inclined to bias my judgments along a predetermined line of purpose and according to a private set of values ?

2. What are the social factors general to my time which I am probably not aware of and which need to be made specific in order that this research may not be warped by a purpose and value peculiar to this immediate instant of time ?

3. What are the specific scientific purposes and values according to which this research is to be conducted ?

4. How can I be aware of changes in purpose and value in any and all of the above areas during the period of the research ? [1]

The Place of Values in Psycho-social Research.

Values are implicit in method. They come to the fore in every research situation, and the failure to consider them fully has led to much sterility in past research where a clinging belief in naïve objectivity has allowed all sorts of subjective bias to creep in. But the matter goes further than this, since psycho-social research of whatever kind is inevitably telic, hence purpose likewise must be considered.

Research which has reform in mind, and allows purpose and concomitant values to remain unstated, merely leaves the social situation where it was before, since it is primarily in the interplay of values and purposes that qualitative change is emergent. Thus an objective statement of research purposes [2] and values dismisses at once the possibility of " scientific disinterestedness " and " idle curiosity " in psycho-social research.

If the research agent makes an explicit statement of the scientific purposes and values held in the research and makes an equal endeavour to become aware of the forms of social and personal conditionings to which he is subject, and attempts to keep aware of these during the research, it is probable that he is doing all he can to bring to the

---

[1] In the above discussion it has been assumed that the reader is familiar with the main points of the dynamic psychologies called " Behaviourism," " Psycho-analysis," and that branch of Social Psychology dealing with attitudes and prejudices.

[2] To be considered in following chapter.

fore the subjective elements liable to affect his research judgment.[1]

But a statement of values, held consciously or unconsciously, is not alone sufficient ; consideration must also be given to the values inherent in the situation being studied.

Values, considered as judgments placed upon one's own or others' activities, are derived from needs, wants, and desires—the dynamic forces in behaviour. When needs, wants, and desires reach the level of release, that is, become the motivating components in actual conduct, values have already become intertwined. He who wants something, wants it because he believes the object of his want will be of value to him. At this point, no consideration needs to be directed toward intrinsic values ; it is important to note merely that valuing of some sort has already taken place. (Considerable difficulty in reasoning about values might be averted if the verb form " to value " were used instead of the noun " value.")

Since needs, wants, desires, and purposes as representative goals of human conduct are conditioned by physical, social, and psychological environments, as well as by the biological individual, it happens that natural groupings tend to arise. Using descriptive terms for the varieties of human experience, we may then formulate, for purposes of convenience, categories of value. Thus, for committees consisting of employees and employers in a given industry, we may say that the values to be

---

[1] This treatment skirts around the probable need for a psycho-analytical interpretation of all people engaged in psycho-social research as a digression too lengthy for present consideration.

discovered are those emanating from the various interests involved. The employer, let us say, has an interest in making his business show profits. Employees have an interest in securing the highest possible wage. Is there to be found a way in which a joint committee, in which both interests are represented, may deal with values which are, in this case, economic ? If, for example, joint committees become so expensive in terms of time lost from employment, and do not compensate for this apparent loss by some other economic contribution, is it not fair to state that the net result, from the point of view of economic value, is negative ? Merely to raise this question signifies the complexity of the problem of values, since it becomes patent at once that some industries might be prepared to absorb the economic loss involved in joint committees, providing other values are conserved. For example, the management might recognize joint committees as costly, and still continue their use on the ground that the committees prevented frictions latent with far greater, although potential, economic loss. In a situation such as this, however, the time might come when the economic cost of committees would endanger net profits, and at this point a choice would need to be made between immediate profit and probable instability of the working force.

For any given situation there is, then, a cluster of values the various items of which must somehow represent consistency, if not unity. Before proceeding with our argument, it may, therefore, be advisable to propose an arbitrary set of values appropriate for joint committees in industry.

Economic values arising from the interest of the employer to maintain a profitable business, and from the employee's interest in securing the highest possible wage.

Technical values arising from the interest of the employer to make the most efficient use of materials, and from the employee's interest in workmanship.

Social values arising from the employer's interest in sustaining a stable, co-operative working force, and from the employee's interest in status, prestige, and self-respect through group representation.

Control values arising from the employer's interest in regulating work with a minimum of friction, and from the employee's interest in self-direction, self-fulfilment, autonomy.

Responsibility values arising from the employer's interest in dispersing a sense of accountableness for quality of work, quantity of output, and from employee's interest in promotion.

Educative values (this term is added because of the fact that committee procedure may, in itself, be considered as a form of learning), arising from the employer's interest in knowledge as an asset to the worker and the company, and from the employee's interest in self-development.

Some such array of values, then, is inherent in the industrial relations as existing, and to which the research agent makes his approach. The values are there to be discovered and to be brought to the foreground, and this is accomplished by means of techniques interfused with the Personal, Social, and Scientific values of the research agent. An abstract, categorical statement of values is of little importance. These must be stated in terms of method ; that is, wherever there is research, values come to the fore. A discussion of values in this particular research will therefore be distributed throughout the section on Technique. What is important, what we wish to emphasize, is that no statement of epistemology and method in social science can be complete, or even valid, without treating of purpose and value.

Following upon self-awareness comes the necessity for the scientific observer to " live into " his situation. From the moment he begins observing a social situation, he exerts an influence upon the participants, and in turn upon the situation itself. Disavowal of such influence leads merely to misinterpretations and false constructions. If, as Dewey appears to insist,[1] truth about phenomena consists of what intelligence does to the phenomena, then the closer the observer can come to his situations, the more truth will be revealed. This assumption, simple as it may sound, leads to important methodological considerations. If the observer comes candidly so near his situation as to exert an influence upon it, he can no longer presume to be studying a static situation ; he is then driven to the utilization of instruments which are capable of perceiving an *evolving situation* ; his method becomes, not photographic, but cinematographic. To perceive one's self as moving along with a situation, and at the same time as observer of its significant events, is

[1] *The Quest for Certainty*, chapter on the " Naturalization of Intelligence."

not a simple task ; it creates a sound demand for new sensibilities, as well as new techniques.   At this point, the " detective " method reveals its disutility ; to " live into " (Spengler's term, " *erfühlen*," [1] or the alternate German word, " *einfühlen*," are more expressive), a social situation contradicts the assumption that an observer may discover the important facts concerning social processes by remaining detached, externalized.

[1] *Decline of the West*, p. 105.

CHAPTER VIII

THE RESEARCH SITUATION AND THE RESEARCH
PURPOSE

" Consciousness is not a substance but a relation—the
relation between the living organism and the environment
to which it specifically responds ; of which its behaviour is
found to be this or that constant function : or, in other words,
to which its purposes refer. . . . In short, those objects or
aspects toward which we respond, of which our purposes are
functions—these are the contents of consciousness."
            —EDWIN HOLT in *The Freudian Wish.*

IN the foregoing chapter we have been particularly
concerned with the epistemological problem of social
research. Social reality, we have said, consists of an
admixture of both objective and subjective elements.
Our chief aim has been to point out how the subjective
elements intrude themselves into the research situation.
It was our contention that values, which are subjective
interpretations of events and qualities, cannot be eliminated from the social research equation and that
therefore it becomes necessary, not merely to take these
into account, but in some manner to include them candidly
as significant aspects of social reality. We suggested that
this might be done by certain intentional conditionings
on the part of the research agent, especially in the
cultivation of certain varieties of self-awareness, and in
acquiring the capacity to " live into " social situations.
It now becomes our task to explain how the research
purpose, that is, the complex of motivations and incentives

which activate the research agent, affects the research situation.

Perhaps a summary statement of comparison between the older conception of social research and the one which we are here setting forth may be useful as an introductory explanation of our argument :

OLDER CONCEPTION	NEWER CONCEPTION
1. Research agent must be free from social and personal purpose ;	1. Research agent must accept the fact of his purposes and proceed to their clarification ;
2. Research agent should cultivate the habit of detachment and disinterestedness ;	2. Research agent should cultivate those qualities of self-awareness which will allow him to take his interests into account ;
3. Research agent should, in so far as possible, keep himself external to the research situation ;	3. Research agent should acquire the capacity to " live into " the research situation ;
4. Research agent should, in so far as possible, exclude his sense of values.	4. Research agent should candidly include his values, as well as values as found in the research situation.

It should be remarked that the above comparison points toward *social* research and not toward all varieties of investigation. Certainly, there are varieties of physical and biological research in which the qualities of disinterestedness and externalization are essentially more realizable. But our reiterated contention is that these various ways of remaining " outside " the situation are not in any sense possible in social research. Before proceeding in our analysis of the rôle of purpose in social research we shall, therefore, and perhaps at the expense of repetition, summarize our objections to the older, naïve positivism in the social sciences :

(a) The presumed disinterestedness which is claimed for the physical and biological sciences is utterly impossible when one human being studies other human beings and their interrelationships.

(b) The varieties of social facts which can be observed and correlated by methods adapted from the physical and biological sciences are relatively crude and for the most part unimportant.

(c) Thus far, social scientists have made more valuable contributions to the understanding of human interrelationships by means of deductive and intuitive insights than through quantitative measurements. [1]

(d) All sciences (as well as all phenomena) are in one sense natural, but human beings bear a relationship to nature which differs in significant ways from that of other objects and organisms, and it

[1] This statement is not to be understood as an argument for the continuation of trust in insight and intuition, but merely to indicate that whatever is lively and stimulating in the social sciences has thus far resulted from individual reflections and not from scientific method. Auguste Comte, the so-called " father " of modern sociology, is, of course, primarily responsible for the positivist emphasis. He believed in the possibility of a Social Physics. His colleague, Saint-Simon, believed, on the other hand, in Social Dynamics. The estrangement which separated them as friends and thinkers followed upon this divergence. Comte wanted to build a new society by the slow methods of scientific analysis whereas Saint-Simon wished to proceed directly toward reconstruction relying upon his intuitions and ideals. We do not suggest in the above statement that Saint-Simon was right and Comte wrong ; on the contrary, it appears to us that the main contention of Comte was correct, but that both he and his followers have been naïve and superficial in its interpretation and application, and because of this, more vitality still resides in those who, like Saint-Simon, have reasoned from intuition and in terms of rough approximations to underlying human purposes. We do not, however, believe that the Saint-Simons will ever be wholly superseded in the social sciences. Our aim is to find a validifying corrective for intuitive social dynamics in the form of a method which is in itself so far social as to include the intuitive and the subjective elements in social relationships.

is this qualitative difference which creates the necessity for a methodology which is more than naïvely " natural."

(e) One of the significant differences in man's relation to nature emanates from his psychic and social dynamic ; this, the telic aspect of man's conduct, proceeds from subjective sources ; individual behaviour and collective direction are both dominated by wishes, values, drives, desires, and purposes ; any scientific method, therefore, which aims to reveal significant facts concerning social phenomena must be one which is inclusive of these subjective elements.[1]

The research experiment upon which this volume is based was an attempt to carry the positive aspect of the above assumptions into practice. We assumed, for example, that two persons who had both been related to economic and industrial studies, and who had been involved in prolonged discussions of their implications, could not suddenly divest themselves of their interests, values, and purposes. Consequently, we began by viewing the total research situation in this manner :

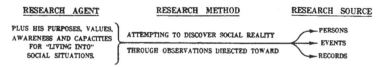

RESEARCH AGENT	RESEARCH METHOD	RESEARCH SOURCE
PLUS HIS PURPOSES, VALUES, AWARENESS AND CAPACITIES FOR "LIVING INTO" SOCIAL SITUATIONS.	ATTEMPTING TO DISCOVER SOCIAL REALITY THROUGH OBSERVATIONS DIRECTED TOWARD	PERSONS EVENTS RECORDS

Research purpose in the agent furnishes the setting within which the total research situation evolves. For

[1] Psychology and physiology may, of course, reduce all of these psychic and social elements in subjectivity to objective entities and processes, but this goal is still far off, and there are good reasons for believing that it may never be a wholly realizable consummation.

each type of research situation there arises a qualitative relatedness between the research agent and each of the elements in the total situation. It is this qualitative relatedness, dominated by purpose, which makes of the research situation an affair of such delicate and subtle proportions. The above diagram, consequently, becomes an over-simplification of the total research situation ; it appears as if purpose were restricted to an attribute of the research agent, whereas it is our contention that purpose modifies the research method, the quality of relatedness between the agent and his fact-sources, and is indeed the controlling factor in the total situation. Ordinarily, research method is regarded as an independent constant within the research situation ; most theorists contend that the subject in research may vary and that the object of research is also a variable, but they maintain that method remains constant no matter who uses it or upon whatever objects it is focused. But it is precisely this dogma of research which we aim to criticize by pointing out that purpose is an all-pervading influence in every ongoing research situation considered as a whole.

In terms of the above modifications it is, perhaps, most logical from our point of view to depict the total research situation as follows :

Research Agent : Utilizing techniques : In Relation to Fact-source

With Research Purpose as the Pervasive Source of Variability throughout the total situation.

This equation, allowing for the element of purpose, and consequent variability throughout the research situation, may appear to make of research method nothing more than the by-product of an individual research agent's personality.   If research method does not constitute a constant, where is one to look for reliability of facts ? The appropriate reply to this query is :   How does one at present discriminate between degrees of reliability of facts ?   If, for example, as it sometimes happens, two research agents, each presuming to have eliminated his purposes, and each using standard methods of research, arrive at conclusions which are diametrically opposed, is it not true that observers impute the difference to purpose or bias ?   Our contention is that reliability of fact will increase in proportion to the inclusion of purpose, not its fictitious exclusion.

With the above modifications of our equation in mind, it may now forward our discussion if we propose that all social research situations normally fall into one of the three following major patterns, namely :

(1) Situations in which the chief quality of relatedness is that which exists between a research agent and another person, or other persons ; such situations may be called *person-to-person* relationships.

(2) Situations in which the chief quality of relatedness is that which exists between a research agent and ongoing events ; such situations may be called *person-to-event* relationships.

(3) Situations in which the chief quality of relatedness is that which exists between a research agent and recorded data ; such situations may be called *person-to-record* relationships.

Research purpose enters into all of these situational patterns but becomes peculiarly important with respect to Number 1, namely, in person-to-person equations. The person who is being used as a fact-source, unfortunately for so-called pure research, also brings his purposes into the situation. In the case of management representatives in industry, for example, it was soon found that these persons were invaluable as fact-sources, but it was also discovered that they were, for the most part, devoid of research purpose. Indeed, whatever purposes they brought into the situation were of the operative-efficiency type and were hence likely to run counter to the research purposes. These men were accustomed to executive-situations, that is, situations in which facts are either taken for granted or referred to technologists. Their chief impulse was " to get things done " and, obviously, time spent on meticulous considerations of committee details did not appear to them as particularly helpful. In general, it may be said that the two sets of purposes as revealed in this study appeared as follows :

RESEARCH PURPOSE :

To discover how joint committees in employee representation operate ;

To learn the extent to which joint committees served educational ends ;

To discover the nature of committee process, or conference procedure employed in joint committees ;

To compare employee representation with trade unionism ;

To experiment with varieties of techniques of research.

MANAGEMENT PURPOSE :

To know how to " run " joint committees ;

To know how to operate employee representation in such manner as to make trade unionism unnecessary ;

To learn how to utilize joint committees as means for disseminating company information;

To discover methods for keeping interest in joint committees alive ;

To acquire methods of conference procedure which would permit management representatives, especially chairmen, to keep ahead of employees with respect to needs, requests, et cetera.

H

It will be seen at once that the above purposes are not merely different but are actually divergent ; the two main concerns of the research agents, namely, conference method as an educational procedure, and research technology, were not shared by management representatives ; on the other hand, some of the purposes found in management representatives were, in reality, headed in a direction opposite to the purposes of the research agents. This is not an unusual situation in social research ; wherever the facts are less than obvious it often occurs that unrevealed and divergent purposes are the factors which tend to conceal reality.[1]

What is to be done in view of divergent purposes ? Denial and escape is an easy way of dismissing a problem of this nature, but it is also a way which falsifies facts. Our procedure led in the opposite direction : we frankly admitted the existence of divergent purposes and then proceeded toward corrective formulæ. The clue to these formulæ is this : Any procedure which will tend to render purposes less static, more flexible, will also tend to lessen divergence. With this clue in mind, we approached the problem of divergent purposes by instigating exchanges which would :

(a) Clarify the purposes of management and of the research agents.

[1] Occasionally one hears of social research originating in the desire of a group, organization, or institution to be investigated ; in such instances it would seem that divergent purposes (as between the research agent and the research source) could not exist. But, familiarity with a number of such " requested " studies leads to the conclusion that even under these circumstances divergent purposes emerge ; indeed, there is at least one record of research of this type which failed completely because of the inability of participants to reconcile their divergent purposes.

(b) Indicate ways in which even preliminary research results might impinge upon and reinforce management's operative-efficiency purposes.

(c) Challenge management purposes by critical examinations of their preconceived values.

Each of these procedures, when appropriately utilized, accomplished two results, namely : (a) it reduced purposes to more flexible terms, and (b) it revealed convergent elements in purposes which were initially conceived as divergent. Wherever convergence of purposes took place the research went beyond superficial levels, and conversely, where purposes remained divergent and inflexible the facts discovered were relatively of little importance.

The Quality of Relatedness influences the Quality of Result.

Relatedness, being the qualitative position of the research agent in a total research situation, varies with each pattern-type of situation. In the above three type-patterns of situation it will be observed that the research agent in each case comes into contact with a research source ; his motive in establishing contact is to elicit information. But a different kind or mode of contact appears for each type. The manner in which these differences occur may be illustrated by indicating what actually happens in each instance, for example :

(1) When the research agent confronts another person (fact-source) the mode of contact is that of communication or interaction ; the media of communication are words, sentences, gestures, grimaces, moods of attentiveness or inattentive-

ness, et cetera.   In short, communication is conditioned by both persons as physiological organisms who see, hear, smell, touch, hold opinions, are motivated by attitudes, use language symbols for expressing ideas, et cetera.

Thus, in person-to-person situations the quality of relatedness depends primarily upon progressive interactions between research agent and another person (fact-source) unimpeded by blockings, misconceptions, suspicions, and other forms of frustration.

(2) When the research agent confronts an event the mode of contact is that of observation.   The research agent's observations are then conditioned by the acuteness of his sense perceptions, his ideal conceptions, his past experience, and whatever recording devices he may utilize.

Thus, in person-to-event situations the quality of relatedness depends primarily upon the observer's perceptive capacities, plus his ability to remain apart from communication as an influence in the event.

(3) When the research agent confronts a record of past events the mode of contact is that of inference ; whatever the observer infers from the record is conditioned by his first-hand acquaintance with similar events gained through situations 1 and 2, his reading habits, his ability to make discriminations, his insight with respect to meanings, and the adequacy of the record.

Thus, in person-to-record situations the quality of relatedness depends primarily upon the research agent's capacity to reconstruct past events through interpretation of derivative descriptions.

The research agent and the research source are not separate and independent variables ; on the contrary,

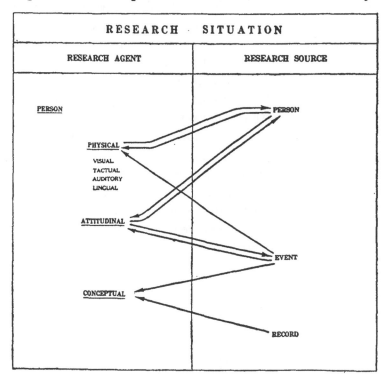

they are interdependent variables, interacting units constituting, together with method, the total research situation. When research techniques are still further refined it will become possible to view these units as consisting of still smaller parts; it will then be seen that interaction between a research agent and each of the three types of research source proceeds according to certain gradients; in the person-to-person relationship, for example, each individual's physical traits and capacities will condition the interacting process, whereas in person-to-record situations conceptual procedures will become more important. Research has not, obviously, reached this degree of refinement, but it may be appropriate to point out how these gradients appear to operate. The diagram below may serve this end.

The quality of the research agent's cognition will vary with respect to the dominant gradient in each research situation. Likewise, the subjective probabilities in each situation will vary with respect to the quality of cognition as conditioned by one or another gradient in the interacting process. Illustrations of such subjective probabilities, taken from experience in the present study, will serve to indicate how subjective elements enter each of the three types of research situation :

	Response in Relation to Purpose :	Subjective Probabilities :
1. In the Person-to-Person Situation :	Response may be to some item in the situation extraneous to the research purpose : — to the interviewer's bodily form ; — to the interviewer's language, or terminology ; — to some item in his own assimilated background called forth by the interviewer, et cetera.	The irrelevant response of the interviews may be due to : — a wish for delay ; — lack of comprehension ; — feeling of insecurity ; — resistances caused by lack of faith in research ; — resistances caused by real lack of desire (motivation) to comprehend, et cetera.

2. In the Person-to-Person Event Situation :	Observer is likely to : — respond to some gradient in the event because of emotional identification with that fraction. Participants in the event (in the case of a committee, *e.g.*) are likely to : — respond to the observer instead of to the dynamics of the event ; — engage in " playing to the galleries " responses, thus falsifying the situation, et cetera.	The research agent : — is apt to impute so much importance to a gradient as to miss or warp the total situation ; — is apt to develop " blind-spots " for all items which do not correspond with his emotional identifications ; — is apt to interpret a " playing - to - the - galleries " response on the part of participants in such manner as to misconstrue the total situation, et cetera.
3. In the Person-to-Record Situation :	Observer responds to : — data already condensed and refined ; — verbal symbols detached from behaviouristic situations ; — observation of recorded data is usually accompanied by lowered attention, fractional response, and selectivity dominated by the research purpose.	The research agent : — supplies meanings of his own when record is incomplete ; — assumes that reliability attaches to written documents and proceeds with unwarranted assurance ; — is likely to regard his own interpolations of records as having validity, whereas each step away from raw data increases fallibility, et cetera.

A Corrective Formula for Error.

Our main thesis in Chapters VII and VIII consists of various ways of stating the problem of social relativity. The facts which social scientists presume to discover and announce are, from our point of view, relative to such a degree and in such numerable ways as to make the application of naïve scientific method unsuitable. In the combination of techniques of research which we have utilized and which are described in the concluding section of this volume will be found our formula for correcting error. We do not assume that absoluteness of fact is possible but rather that relative knowledge may be made more reliable if certain refinements of research methodology are utilized. Reliability, however, does not reside in any one technique ; on the contrary, facts discovered by a single technique are especially to be mistrusted. Social statistics, for example, are not trustworthy unless the facts enumerated and collated have been examined by some other technique which is qualitatively distinguished from mathematics.

The techniques which we have employed in the present study, together with our fact-expectations for each, are :

TECHNIQUE	EXPECTATION
1. Interviewing : (Informal conversation or formalized interview conducted by the outside observer consisting of verbal interactions).	May reveal attitudes, conceptions, philosophies, opinions, etc., of those engaged in and responsible for committee operations.
2. Participant observation of an event : (Observations made by a member of the committee and checked later by outside observers).	May reveal underlying interests, conflicts, motivations, etc., which an outside observer could not detect.
3. Direct observation of an event : (An observer present at a committee meeting).	May reveal the committee as a moving reality indicating fractional information regarding committee processes, personality interplay, et cetera.
4. Case Study Analysis : (Analysis of an ongoing sequence of committee events related to a single problem).	May reveal more detailed knowledge of committee processes than is possible when an isolated committee session is observed ; may also present facts concerning the " whole ", facts which are likely to be lost in isolated observations

TECHNIQUE	EXPECTATION
5. Charting : (Graphic presentation of certain aspects of committee processes).	May reveal analytical features of the flow of interaction in such manner as to illumine some of the quantitative and qualitative features of participation.
6. Quantitative Analysis : Selection of some item in the whole which is pertinent and relevant and which may be correlated with some other item or items in the total problem).	May constitute a quantitative check on qualitative interpretations derived from one or more of the other techniques.

These six ways of discovering social facts constitute for us the technology of research method and are consequently called techniques. It is our belief that combinations of these six techniques will give assurance of greater reliability than might be expected from any one by itself. The ideal procedure would be, obviously, a composite use of all six techniques.

Wherever the research agent looks and whatever information he tabulates, the result is certain to be a mixture of subjective and objective elements. The reliability of his data will increase in proportion to his admission and utilization of the subjective elements in each research situation. He can eliminate the subjective only by denials of purpose, arbitrary selections of facts, and the employment of techniques so naïve in conception as to make final results both untrustworthy and unusable.

PART IV

EXPERIMENTING WITH SOCIAL TECHNIQUES
AND DEVICES

PART FOUR

EXPERIMENTING WITH SOCIAL TECHNIQUES AND DEVICES

MOST treatises dealing with the problems of social research appear to make the assumption that social reality may be revealed by any one of a number of fact-finding techniques. We postulate the opposite assumption, namely, that all varieties of technique, in so far as they reveal different aspects of reality, are necessary for any given research project. The technology of research is a composite of all available fact-finding devices utilized in conjunction with each other and as checks upon each other. The research situation consists of the research agent, his techniques, and the research source. Stated as a relationship between the research agent and the research source the research situation presents three basic forms, namely :

Person (research agent) to *Person* (as involved in the phenomena to be investigated).

Person (research agent) to *Event* (as immediately observed).

Person (research agent) to *Record* (the event as history).

Each basic form of the research situation represents potentialities of fact-finding not to be found in any one or both of the other two. The ensuing chart (to be found on pages 126 and 127) will indicate how the separate techniques and devices for fact-finding are related to the basic research forms and also what kinds of knowledge each may be expected to reveal.

CHAPTER IX

(Basic Form : The Person-to-Person Relationship)

THE first of the following series of techniques aims to show how the discourse on method in the preceding chapters may be applied in that most pertinent form of person-to-person relationship, namely, the interview. Conversation, as a person-to-person relation, also has its place in research, but the chief distinction between an interview and conversation lies in this : the purpose, even if unexpressed and unfelt, in conversation is primarily better acquaintance or mere exchange of experience, while in the interview, a more specific objective is essential, and in order to maintain a valid relation between interviewer and interviewee, this objective must be known, expressed. But these two forms of person-to-person response are both used in the sort of collaborative research which this report describes. For example, in the initial or preliminary interview it often becomes necessary in view of certain resistances, to keep the specific objectives in the background until conversation can pave the way for better acquaintance.

Fact-finding, Fact-eliciting, and Fact-discovering.

The process of " finding " facts involves a naïve presupposition, namely, that the facts are there, that they

SOCIAL RESEARCH VIEWED AS A SET OF
AGENT AND THE

The Person-to-Person Relationship   *The Person-to-Event*

INTERVIEWING	OBSERVING (Participant)	OBSERVING (Direct)
1. Knowledge of the structural features of joint committees and committee procedures. 2. Attitudes regarding committee functions, processes, results, and values. 3. Opinions regarding committee functions, processes, results, and values. 4. Conceptions of committees, their functions, etc., as conditioned by their general business philosophy. 5. Knowledge of the extent to which Management representatives are aware of the need for research in this area, and how far their general purposes with respect to committees may be combined with the research agents' purposes.	1. The committee session as unique situation. 2. The rôle of the chairman. 3. Personality differences. 4. Quantity and quality of participation. 5. The rôle of the representatives. 6. Characteristic reactions and interactions. 7. Cycles of tempo and tone.	1. Physical factors : — Room ; — Seating ; etc. 2. Situation. 3. Pre-conference factors. 4. Time : (a) Spent on committee session ; (b) Required for single item of business. 5. Subject - matter introduced. 6. Participation. 7. Overt, non-verbal behaviour. 8. Conference progression. 9. Chairman's conduct and characteristic modes. 10. Tempo of interaction 11. Treatment of difference. 12. Conclusions reached.

RELATIONSHIPS BETWEEN THE RESEARCH
RESEARCH SOURCE

Relationship   *The Person-to-Record Relationship*

CASE ANALYSIS	CHARTING	STATISTICS
1. Chronology of significant events : (a) Within a conference setting ; (b) Outside conference setting. 2. Interpretation of significant events considered in sequences. 3. Interpretation of evolution of case in terms of : (a) The nature of the problem ; (b) Interest-distance on the main issue ; (c) Use of facts ; (d) Treatment of differences ; (e) Blockings other than differences and interest-distance ; (f) Kinds of conference procedure used at different stages ; (g) Conclusions reached.	1. Detailed analysis of verbal participations in terms of language forms. 2. Person-to-person interactions denoted as units of participation. 3. Conference phases as determined by nodal points in conference progression. 4. Major characteristics of chairman and representatives' behaviour. 5. Range of participation. 6. Quality of participation. 7. Inference of attitude patterns in chairman and representatives.	1. Record of verbal stimuli indicating : (a) Source of initiation ; (b) Subject ; (c) Manner of introducing subject ; (d) Language mode used in initiating subject. 2. Record of organization preparatory to response as indicated by : (a) Implicit individual consideration ; (b) Explicit individual consideration ; (c) Explicit collective consideration. 3. Record of responses as indicated by : (a) Implicit, non-overt, tacit conclusion ; (b) Explicit, overt conclusion.

exist in objective form, or within a set of relations, and that what is needed is an observer sufficiently disinterested to allow his perceptual capacities to function without emotional interference. However true this conception of scientific method may be for the physical sciences, it certainly does not apply to social phenomena. Of course, certain facts are there to be observed, and a degree of disinterestedness will aid in seeing those facts more clearly. But, the facts which may be thus observed are, in most cases, insignificant, or so clearly obvious as to throw no light upon fundamental processes. For example, it is clear, if one is studying a committee as a social phenomenon, that an outside observer could, with only the use of the senses of hearing and sight, find a number of facts ; he would know that there were a certain number of individual human beings participating ; that one of these was acting as leader or chairman ; that some talked a great deal while others remained silent ; that the kind and quality of the talking varied with subjects, et cetera, et cetera. But how significant are such facts for an understanding of the real process going on within the committee ?

Fact-eliciting implies that the pertinent facts are not lying about ready for the observer to record, but, on the contrary, that the most important facts are buried within a social complex ; further, that such facts can only be revealed by a method which is in itself thoroughly social. Only when the interviewer and the interviewee are responding in the interest of a similar, if not an identical, goal can there be an eliciting of facts which is self-validifying. Indeed, it may be said that when those engaged in the social process and those engaged in social investigation have purposes which are confluent, the result of study is not fact-finding, nor alone fact-eliciting, but rather fact-discovery. The detective finds facts by methods of external observation, the news reporter elicits facts, the social scientist may find and elicit facts, but if he is to push his inquiries beneath the top layers of social phenomena, he will need to be a fact-discoverer. Fact-finding is in itself a naïve proceeding and nearly all social studies, which are not merely statistical enumerations of facts presumed by others, or of relations between facts subsumed by the investigator, utilize some method of fact-eliciting. The two most generally employed methods are the questionnaire and the interview. The former was not used in this study but the latter was given considerable emphasis.

Interviewing consists of dialogue, verbal responses between two persons or between several persons. These responses, while verbal in an objective sense, are conditioned by a number of other factors, some of which are subjective and some objective. For example, the physical surroundings in which an interview takes place influence the procedure significantly. In some of the older texts on applied psychology one may find references indicating methods for controlling these environmental factors ; some of these writers gave directions for seating, flow of light, et cetera, with a view of placing one party to an interview at a disadvantage. Such procedures are, obviously, unjustified. But if the interview is to be used as a specialized tool on psycho-social research, attention must be directed toward even such seemingly unimportant

I

elements as are involved in seating arrangements, comfort, light, et cetera.

The initial objective of the investigators, in this case, was to secure permission from officials of various industrial enterprises to study the processes of their joint employee-management committees. But this objective included two additional goals ; it was desired to secure this permission (*a*) in such manner as to include the officials as interested observers of the investigation, if not as collaborators, and (*b*) in such manner as to make a continuation of the study possible for those within the organization. The major objective is not unlike that of most interviews in which the interviewer uses the interview as a method for securing something, either as a privilege, or concession from someone else. The associated objectives, however, constitute a new hypothesis for interviewing, and in one sense become more important than the major objective. If, for example, the interview is so conducted as to gain permission for study but at the same time isolates those concerned with the industry from those conducting the investigation, research at once slips back into its old groove ; it becomes a method of external abstraction. The triple aspect of the initial interview's objective may be portrayed as follows :

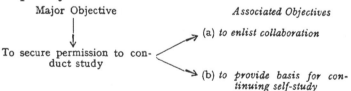

Before proceeding to devise an interview technique using these objectives, the prospective interviewer will be obliged to anticipate, in so far as possible, the general mind-set of management officials when confronted with a request of this sort. The responsible official will, in all likelihood, enter the situation with both positive and negative attitudes and opinions, and the interviewer, if he is committed to a co-operative principle, will take both what is favourable and what is unfavourable into account. In the present study it was found that the negative and positive attitudes encountered were approximately the following :

POSITIVE ATTITUDES	NEGATIVE ATTITUDES
(a) Concern for committee success.	(a) General suspicion toward the outsider.
(b) Generalized interest in research.	(b) Scepticism regarding the possibility of measuring committee functioning.
(c) Generalized need for indices of measurements.	(c) Normal resistance to self-analysis.
(d) Receptivity due to former contact with persons known to the investigators.	(d) Reliance upon company morale rather than technical committee process.
(e) Committee studies already undertaken by members of personnel staff.	(e) Reluctance to engage upon an investigation the results of which promise to increase one's labours.

Obviously, success in the investigation varied with respect to the force of the negative attitudes, and with respect to the ability of the investigators to overcome negativism, or to transmute negativism into positivism. The degree of success covered a span beginning with complete and thorough-going mutuality to complete and ultimate failure.

It is safe to say that some of the negative attitudes in even the two most favourable companies were not entirely dispelled until the study was far advanced, and only in one company was there a final assurance that all negativism had disappeared. This fact elevates interviewing to the plane of primary importance, since every step in the progress of the study was interpreted to company officials by means of interviews. Even when the investigators were displaying practical results, results which obviously aided in weakening resistance, the method of presentation utilized was the interview.

Types of Interviews.

Since each interview is preconceived in terms of a specific objective, it follows that interviews tend to fall into classes, with purpose as the chief factor of definition. Analysis of the interview records resulting from the present study reveals at least four types :

(1) *The initial, preliminary, or approach interview.*

As stated above, this initial interview, while conceived in simple terms as an attempt to secure permission to conduct a study, includes also the other two objectives, namely, that of continuing collaboration, and possible self-study in the future. But still further removed from these objectives is the more general one of creating favourable attitudes. It is at this point that the interviewer needs to be constantly aware of the potentially unfavourable attitudes which may motivate the interviewee. Three general rules may be adduced for this initial step in interviewing :

(*a*) Only a few relevant facts need to be elicited ; too many would tend to confuse both the interviewer and the person being interviewed.

(*b*) Main attention should be placed upon understanding, that is, upon the effort to make sure that possible misconceptions are eliminated.

(*c*) Emphasis should be placed upon the request being made, but in such manner as to enable the interviewee to see its significance in a number of directions.

The difference between success and failure in the initial interview is often determined by previous contacts. For example, if the interviewer comes with an introduction, or with sponsorship, the way is cleared for a quick approach to the main request; on the other hand, if the interviewer labours under the necessity of going through the various stages of acquaintance, much more time will be required, and the initial interview may in fact be stretched out over a large number of individual sessions. This happened to be the case in the present study with all save one company. And, as indicated above, in at least one company the interviewers failed to complete even the purpose of the initial interview, although in this case separate sessions were held up to the number of eight.

(2) *The enlisting, informing, reciprocating interview.*

Once the initial stage is past and favourable attitudes exist in sufficient degree to warrant advance, the interviewer finds himself under obligations to explain his project. Difficulties of many varieties enter at this point : the investigator, for example, is likely to interpret his research in technical, academic language ;

the practical-minded executive in industry is not merely unfamiliar with this terminology, but he has definite misgivings concerning those who employ it. Abstract concepts are likely to enter these early discussions, or what is even more damaging, terms may be used in two or more different ways. One rule may be accepted, namely, that the interviewee is not likely to proceed much further with the study if he finds that he does not understand the language of the investigators. On the other hand, new concepts need to be introduced, and it is the investigator's function to allow these to enter the discussion without formality ; also it is his function to see that these new terms are interpreted in the light of experience-patterns likely to be found in industrial executives. In short, enough information concerning the nature of the project should be introduced to enlist interest and curiosity, but not enough to induce feelings of bewilderment or inferiority.

One general deduction made by the investigators as a result of their experience may be stated as follows : In so far as this phase of interviewing is intended to enlist the interviewee's interest and curiosity, and at the same time lead him forward in an understanding of the project, it must be so conducted as to allow for reciprocal information-giving. If the interviewer begins with a rigid plan to which he adheres without modification, he may secure assent for his project but he will not carry the interviewee along in succeeding steps. In short, the interviewer must be prepared to change his postulates in terms of the kinds of facts which the interviewee announces and in which he has faith. In the present study, for example, it was soon learned that certain industrial executives were opposed to direct observations of committees while in session. Their reasons for this position turned out to be sound, but if insistence at this point had been expressed by the investigators, no further progress could have been expected. What actually happened was this: the investigators revamped their hypotheses and their methods to allow for this reservation.

(3) *The " check-up " or collaborating interview.*

After interview stages 1 and 2 had been consummated, it was found necessary to conduct a continuing series of interviews over a long period of time for the express purpose of keeping the officials of the company in a collaborating mood. It is at this point that the investigators begin to bring back facts which they believe to have been discovered. The purpose here is to test these facts, to secure corroboration or correction, but also to give the co-operators an opportunity to share in the project. Check-up interviews were sometimes held with individuals, and at other times with groups. Whenever feasible, co-operators were asked to perform some function allied with the project as a whole. If such a function could be related in a constructive sense to the ongoing tasks of the person, this opportunity was grasped. In several instances employees actually changed their methods of work in the light of facts revealed by the study. In other words, these interviews were conducted in an atmosphere of " working together," as distinguished from the more orthodox method of research in which the investigator's facts were withheld until the time of a final report.

Interviewing Rationale.

In order to simplify and condense our rationalistic premises for the technique of co-operative interviewing we shall present our arguments in the form of direct propositions :

(1) The interviewer needs to be aware at all times of his dual goal, namely, to secure facts, and to keep the fact-giver vitally interested in the procedure.

(2) Co-operative interviewing represents an equation in which a personalized relationship exists between the research agent and the person collaborating in the discovery of facts. (The usual equation— impersonal fact-finder interrogating an impersonal fact-source is frankly discarded.)

(3) Co-operative interviewing requires of the interviewer a capacity for shifting his base without losing sight of his research purpose ; he must take the fact-source (person) wherever he finds him, and proceed from this point to fuller elaboration of the research purpose by means of educational processes.

(4) Co-operative interviewing is based upon the assumption that the results are combinations of objective-subjective facts.[1]

---

[1] The questionnaire as instrument for fact-finding may be utilized at this point for comparative purposes. The research agent who fills in the answers to his questions refrains from making subjective judgments ; he merely tabulates without interpreting meanings and is particularly happy when his answers appear in " yes " or " no "

(5) The co-operative interview allows for a total view since it includes clues furnished by those who actually " live in " the situation under observation, clues which the outside observer might miss.

(6) Co-operative interviewing goes deeper as well as further because it reveals underlying conditioning factors in social situations, such as feelings, attitudes, opinions, et cetera.

(7) The results of co-operative interviewing present themselves as valid, not merely to the research agent, but also to the research source ; when the interviewee is subjected to a one-way type of interview he is always left free to challenge the research agent's interpretation.

From the point of view of the interviewer, whatever techniques and skills are utilized, their primary aim is to release the interviewee, to create for him an atmosphere in which he may talk freely and without constraint. In order to achieve this, the interviewer must put the notion of automatic response out of mind. The interviewer is not merely a recorder of responses ; he is the guide for a process ; his task, once release has been accomplished, is to guide the sequence of response, to hold it in the direction of the project's main objective. The more formal, technical, and scientific the interview appears on the surface, the less release will be secured. The chief art of the interview is to steer a course without awareness

form. What he overlooks, of course, is that his subjective judgments have entered into his questions and consequently are reflected in the answers. He allows subjectivity to enter *via* the back door whereas co-operative interviewing admits subjective elements by the front door.

of maps, compasses, and sextants.   The methodological framework must be there, and must function, but it should not be seen.   Hence, it may be correct to speak of the " technique " of interviewing, but in a very real sense interviewing which is highly successful has already passed its technical phase and has become an art.

An initial interview will now be tested according to all three of the objectives mentioned earlier in the chapter. By condensing the material of an actual interview of this type we may now proceed to conduct such a test.

CONDENSED RECORD OF AN INITIAL INTERVIEW (COMPANY " C ")

Sequence of Subjects Introduced : (" x " and " y " designate the two interviewers)	Responses of Two Interviewees " A " and " B "	Interviewer's Interpretations : in terms of categories of analysis
Queries by " x " regarding structure of employee representation plan in this industry.	Replies readily given and elaborated, consisting of descriptions of Division Committees, Executive Council, and Joint Employee-Management Works Committee.	*Circumjacence :* Mgt.'s conception of emp. rep. as structure.
Queries by " x " and " y " regarding the kinds of problems discussed in these various conference groups.	Response indicated that they all discussed the same sorts of problems ; divisional committees appear most important since they deal with first-hand situations arising in the shops. The other two committees are sources of appeal. The chief subject coming before all committees is wage adjustment.	*Interaction :* Mgt.'s interpretation of problems discussed by committees. *Circumjacence :* Mgt.'s conception of importance as between two committees.
Queries by " x " and " y " directed toward the underlying conference conceptions of "A" and " B."	" A " believes that voting is not necessary. " B " speaks of the possibility of reaching integrative conclusions in committees. "A" believes that that plan is best in which the fewest number of cases reach conference level.	*Interaction :* Mgt.'s attitude toward voting, toward levels of adjustment, training, etc.

CONDENSED RECORD OF AN INITIAL INTERVIEW (COMPANY " C ")
—*Continued*

Sequence of Subjects Introduced : (" x " and " y " designate the two interviewers)	Responses of Two Interviewees " A " and " B "	Interviewer's Interpretations : in terms of categories of analysis
	"A" believes that that employee representative is best who can induce men to arrive at adjustment without bringing case to committee.	
	"A" believes that no formal training is necessary for committee work.	*Impulsion :* Mgt.'s pride in the stability of its plan.
	"A" states plan has been in operation ten years and appears to be accepted as normal part of the organization.	
	"A" does not believe that : the fact that few employee representatives participate in discussion represents a serious problem.	*Interaction :* Mgt.'s conception of committee process.
" B " asks for permission to visit a joint conference.	"A" replies with a kind but firm negative, adding that a rule had been adopted to stop visiting because of the annoyance this had caused.	(Attitude of restraint toward research agents.)
" x " asks for permission to proceed with his analysis of minutes of previous meetings.	This permission is granted.	(Attitude of confidence toward research agents.)
" y " proposes that it might be useful to organize a small study group of employee and management representatives to discuss conference procedures.	There appeared to be difficulties in the way of such a project, and although neither "A" nor " B " explicitly said so, it seemed that they needed higher authority before making a decision.	(Attitude of interest in proposal but reserve, probably because of lack of adequate authority.)
	" B " suggested that such a group might be organized as a part of the training school.	(Attitude of positive response toward research agents indicated by re-enforcing suggestions.)
	"A" suggested that it might be considered as a part of the management curriculum in the school.	

Composite Interpretation : Analysis of the interviewer's interpretations in the right-hand column in terms of the three objectives of the initial interview reveals : that the major objective (to secure information to conduct study) was only partially realized ; (*a*) that considerable resistance toward collaboration existed ; (*b*) that the interviewees were not sufficiently motivated to respond with complete favour to the notion of continuing study within the industry ; (*c*) that the interviewees were prepared to furnish unrefined information concerning joint committees in their industry.

Interviewing and the Categories of Psycho-social Research.

Interviewing is the primary technique for revealing attitudes, opinions, preconceptions, and values. These, as has already been indicated, play an important rôle in the intermixture of all social facts and social situations ; if left entirely in their subjective setting, these psychic attributes will influence final results in a most invidious manner. And it is these very psychic determinants of social situations which are never revealed in records or in the " outsider's " survey of events. One recognizes these more subtle factors in interviewing, and in the give and take of responses one is able to test and recheck at once ; a request for restatements, repetitions, or rephrasings often furnishes the clarified meaning. Thus, one executive in an early interview dropped a casual remark concerning the futility of democracy ; he was obviously revealing his sense of values, and although the remark was not wholly relevant at the moment, it served to refashion succeeding interviews until his meaning, in so far as related to joint committees, was entirely clear.

The first of our four categories of research, namely, *Impulsion* (Chapter III) includes the notion of purpose. Our desire was to learn as much as possible concerning the purposes which employers had in mind when initiating their employee representation plans, together with their purposes as evolved during experience. At this point the interviewer was obliged to sustain a sensitive mood with respect to such items as (*a*) the quality of enthusiasm, or lack of enthusiasm, as expressed by the interviewee ; (*b*) the amount of time, and degree of patience, the interviewee was willing to devote to a difficult question related to purposes ; (*c*) the kind of initiative, or lack of initiative, which this company has exercised in refining its plan (as distinguished from mere imitativeness).

Purpose, in employee representation, is however, twofold, of the employer and the employee. Interviewing was also utilized as the means of discovering how far the employers were including employee purpose in their reflections about joint committees. How, in fact, does management conceive of the worker's purpose ? Do they actually desire to know what lies at the bottom of the employee's wishes and wants, or are they primarily interested in cultivating his loyalty to the company ? Does management aim at continuance of the duality between employers and employees, or do they conceive of the joint committee as a means for promoting a unifying purpose ?

Circumjacence, as defined in Chapter IV, includes those conditioning factors which to a greater or lesser degree influence the quality of work which joint committees are capable of performing. Chief among these factors is, of course, employer psychology. What does management want these committees to do ? How far does management conceive of the joint committee as structurally flexible or fixed ? Does management view such factors as committee methods, voting procedures, caucuses, rules of order, et cetera, as guides to a dynamic process of human relations, or as static controls ? These are, obviously, subtle elements in the total outlook of management representatives and cannot be revealed by mere guessing. Interviewing was at this point our main resource.

From the beginning to the end of this study our main objective may be said to have been to discover the nature of the actual process or *Interaction* (Chapter V) which goes on in the meetings of joint committees. At this point our main resource for research purposes was the study of records and the observation of committee sessions. We did, however, indirectly, discover other items related to interaction by means of interviewing. For example, we learned indirectly that certain management representatives maintained an attitude toward the so-called " loud-speaker," the employee who talked easily and loudly in committee meetings, and likewise toward the grievance-bearing " crank," and toward other types of employee representatives. These attitudes influenced interaction because they tended to place such type-persons into fixed categories ; the " loud-speaker " and the " crank " were often considered to be nuisances and their contributions might therefore be disregarded by management.

In our attempt to discover the nature of the end-results

of joint committee processes we relied mainly upon records and observations, but we also discovered through interviewing what the principal management attitudes were and how far these conditioned emergence (see Chapter VI). Some management representatives, for example, are satisfied if the joint committee deals with *expository, informative* items in which employers have arrived at a decision which is in turn conveyed to employees through the instrumentality of the joint committee. Others seemed to be eager for committee business which would involve real differences, and which would consequently lead to lively interaction and important decisions. Both attitudes, apparently, tend to influence the quality of end-results possible for joint committees.

From the above it will be seen that interviewing represented an important technique for this study inasmuch as it was utilized in relation to all categories of research. Many of the pertinent facts concerning *impulsion, circumjacence, interaction* and *emergence* were revealed through direct person-to-person interviews. But interviewing is not wholly adequate for social research ; other supplementary techniques are needed, first to act as checks upon facts secured through interviewing, and second, in order to reveal other facts which are of the social process itself, and for which interviewing serves as a secondary fact-source. Before proceeding to the description of these remaining techniques it should be added that interviewing as a tool for social research may be made more reliable if certain procedures are employed. Below will be found an outline depicting a procedure for interview reporting and recording.

The Interview Report.

In order to maintain order within a technique which is so flexible as interviewing, we have prepared a chart to be used by the interviewer, this to be filled in as quickly as possible following the actual interview. This chart consists of five main categories and appears as follows :

A. *Setting.*

Names of Participants.   Date.
Physical conditions.

    Weather.   Place.
    Lighting.
    Heating.   Time of day.
    Ventilation.

What evidence of special planning for the occasion ?

B. *Preliminaries.*

Social atmosphere at beginning.
Kind of greeting. Any formality ?
Did interviewer appear welcome ?
Time limit—was it announced at beginning ?
Was it adhered to ?
What preliminary conversations took place ?
Was the purpose revealed or obscured—preliminary
    conversations ?
Was there any apparent evasion ?
Action—Interaction in the beginning of the inter-
    view.
Initiative by whom ? Responses.

C. *Recording the Interview.*

Interviewer		Interviewee			Inferences
Contribution	Purpose	Facts	Opinions	Overt Behaviour	

D. *Conclusion.*

Social atmosphere at conclusion.

Kind of departure.

Factors influencing the actual conclusion of the interview.

Relations between original purpose of interviewer and actual development and conclusion of the interview.

1. At what point was original purpose side-tracked ?

2. Did interviewee perceive purpose of interviewer ?

(1) Informed by letter.

(2) Direct statement at beginning.

E. *Comments.*

Did the interviewee talk freely ? (Tempo of the process.)

Other comments.

K

Research students appear to be unanimous in the opinion that the procedure of taking direct notes during the interview is a questionable practice.   In a preliminary interview and where both parties are known to each other it is probably advisable to take no notes but to rely upon one's memory for the notation of facts.   If key-words can be fixed in mind at the time, it becomes a simple matter to recall series and sequences of subjects later.   In the preliminary interview it becomes exceedingly important to observe the interviewee's overt behaviour as well as his verbal responses.   His gestures, physical signs, tone of voice, et cetera, furnish a background for the interviewer's questions.   Above all, it must be made clear at this juncture that the interviewee fully understands the purpose of the interview ;   his emotional and physical responses are as valuable here as his oral statements. When research has reached the stage of utilization of the third type of interview it becomes necessary to record direct quotations and to make immediate notations of responses.   At this stage, however, it often happens that formal interviewing technics have been replaced by more informal conversations and discussions.

CHAPTER X

PARTICIPANT OBSERVING AS A TECHNIQUE FOR
PSYCHO-SOCIAL RESEARCH

(Basic Form : The Person-to-Person Relationship)

DIRECT observation of a social event involves at least three specific limitations : (a) the external observer may become a stimulus to the event ; (b) his descriptions of objective factors need to be couched in the simplest of behaviouristic terms (the subjective elements in the interaction, which we believe to be highly important, will be lost to such an observer ; if he attempts to introduce these subjective elements later, he will be forced to utilize a method of general abstraction) ; (c) the conclusions reached by the external observer may be challenged by the participants in an event, and in that circumstance the observer has but one recourse ; he must rest his case upon his reliability as a person, or upon the reliability of his perceiving capacities. He may, of course, attempt verification by allowing other observers to observe similar events (since no two events are identical) and then rest his case upon the collaborated result.

With these limitations in mind we have attempted to find correctives for direct observation.[1] The principal corrective employed in this study is given the name

[1] See *Social Discovery*, by E. C. Lindeman, for an initial interpretation of this technique.

Participant Observation, a technique which may be described in the following terms :

> *Participant Observation* is based on the theory that an interpretation of an event can only be approximately correct when it is a composite of two points of view, the *outside* and the *inside.* Thus the view of the person who was a participant in the event, whose wishes and interests were in some way involved, and the view of the person who was not a participant but only an observer, or analyst, coalesce in one final synthesis.

Participant Observation as utilized in this study proceeded as follows ·

1. A series of interviews was held to acquaint the interested parties with the idea ; to get their permission and finally to sensitize two particular persons who were to be the observers. These two were members of the management group and had been attending the meetings in the past as part of their regular duties.

2. The committee meeting was held ; the participant observers attended, verbatim minutes were kept and a copy sent to the research agents.

3. The research agents prepared an analysis of the meeting with detailed questions to be asked the participant observers.

4. Finally a group interview was held at which the participant observers, as well as several other participants, were present.

The final interpretation of the event is then a composite result of (a) direct observation by the participant observer ; (b) interpretations by the research agents ; (c) reinterpretations of the event following upon reference to the participant observer and other participants. It will be seen that a technique of this sort can only be utilized in social situations where suspicions as between research agents and participants have been dissipated. So long as the gathering and interpretation of social facts is not viewed with sympathy by the participants, the research agent, if he is to proceed at all, must perforce secure his information by whatever external techniques are available.

Participant Observing Illustrated.

In the following cases the participant observer was asked to give special attention to two factors in a coming joint committee session, namely : (a) the chairman's conduct, and (b) conference procedures. Inclusion of the complete data in this case would probably be inadvisable, and consequently we furnish the following :

I. *Some general facts concerning this particular joint committee :*

— the committee consisted of five representatives of Management, and nine representatives of the Employees ;

— the meeting was called as a response to a request coming from the employees who wished to present a specific problem ;

— the chairman of the committee, a Management representative, holds a high position in the company;

— the Employee chairman held a clerical position, slightly higher in rank than that of the other representatives;

— the meeting began at 12:06 p.m. and adjourned at 5:00 p.m.;

— two visitors attended this meeting, both belonging to the technical or managerial staff; they were invited because of their special knowledge pertaining to one of the problems to be discussed at this session;

II. *Sequence and Interpretation of the committee meeting, plus certain questions on conference procedure presented to the participant and the participant observer.*

a	b	c
Sequence of events in the Committee session, as derived from the record.	The Chairman's conduct as derived from interpretations of the record.	Conference procedure questions to be used by research agents in a group interview with the chairman of the committee, the participant observer, and several other Management officials involved in committee operations.
I. Statement of the problem by the Employee Chairman : 1. Employee request for additional holidays : Lincoln's Birthday, Good Friday, Columbus Day, Armistice Day. 2. Arguments in support : (a) Other departments already enjoy these holidays ; (b) Service now dependable ; (c) Other companies' employees now have those days off ; (d) Conditions here not materially different, and management equally capable. 3. E.C. asks that the start be made by granting time off for empls. on the coming Good Friday.		1. This question has been discussed in all district meetings. From this point of view, did the E.C. make the best use of the opinion generated in these prior meetings ? 2. The employee reps. met in caucus before the joint session ; obviously, they were agreed to make this request. Should the E.C. have mentioned at the outset what happened in this previous meeting? 3. What was involved in the E.C.'s reference to equal capacity of mgt. in Pa., New York and New Jersey ? 4. Were the E.C.'s arguments convincing, logically sound ?
II. Rejoinder by the management chairman : 1. Does not disagree with some of fundamental statements of E.C. 2. But problem must be considered in terms of all its factors. 3. Changing working conditions because another company does is not good practice. 4. Problem must be considered in terms of	1. The M.C. was apparently performing the following functions : (a) Factoring out the problem ; (b) Refining the problem ; (c) Reducing the problem to specific local terms ; (d) Rebutting certain arguments of the E.C. ; (e) Justifying mgt. ;	1. Would it have been advisable at this point to: (a) Test the opinion of the group ? (b) To inquire how general the demand is ? (c) To sharpen the problem without answering arguments ? (d) To respond in such manner as to leave his opinion unrevealed ?

a	b	c
Sequence of events in the Committee session, as derived from the record.	*The Chairman's conduct as derived from interpretations of the record.*	*Conference procedure questions to be used by research agents in a group interview with the chairman of the committee, the participant observer, and several other Management officials involved in committee operations.*
II.—*continued* our local situation ; taxes, revenues, service conditions. 5. Our average wage slightly higher than other industries in environment; we must not be too far ahead or behind. 6. Some of our forces may be off on certain holidays without impairing service. 7. Holidays are privileges, not rights. 8. Main question is : What can we do in view of our responsibility to the public ? 9. Practices with respect to holidays differ widely throughout the country. 10. Explanation of New Jersey situation.		(e) To ask for further arguments ? 2. How many negatives and how many positives were included in the M.C.'s rejoinder ? 3. Were his arguments logically sound ? 4. From the point of view of getting the best possible committee process, should the M.C. have voiced the mgts. position in this manner. Rather should not some other mgt. rep. have done it ?
III. At this point the M.C. asked if anyone wished to express disagreement with any of his statements. No responses were forthcoming.	1. The M.C. was here "putting it up to the group." 2. His purpose seemed to be to discover whether or not his points were being accepted or rejected. 3. This was a pause, apparently not for the purpose of precipitating general discussion, but rather for the purpose of testing the effect of his rejoinder.	1. Would it have been advisable at this point to ask for agreement rather than disagreement ? 2. If the M.C. really wanted to reveal differences of attitude and opinion, did he use a method likely to elicit responses ? 3. Since no spontaneous responses were made, would it have been advisable to call on specific persons for expressions of opinion ?

a	b	c
Sequence of events in the Committee session, as derived from the record.	The Chairman's conduct as derived from interpretations of the record.	Conference procedure questions to be used by research agents in a group interview with the chairman of the committee, the participant observer, and several other Management officials involved in committee operations.
IV. The M.C. resumes his remarks : 1. The problem must be discussed in terms of Philadelphia. 2. Better and better service is expected of us. 3. Certain employees in other areas must work on special holidays. 4. Trouble reports are proportional to usage, and we have as many on these days as usual. 5. Other public utilities maintain their services. 6. In N.J. about 75 per cent. of the maintenance force works on these holidays but receives overtime. 7. Some other utilities are more rapid than we are at installations. 8. In view of public demand, we do not have the right to extend our holidays. 9. Mgt. is anxious to give emps. all they can. 10. We were among first to give Saturday afternoons off. 11. So far as evidence goes we believe public wants service on these days. 12. The cost to the Co. would approx. $100,000 if emps. had to work and receive extra pay on these days.	1. For the most part, the M.C. was here making his case against the extension of holidays. 2. He seemed to be attempting to weight the factor of the company's responsibility to the public. 3. He added new facts. 4. He made new comparisons. 5. He continued to justify management. 6. He introduced an entirely new component of the problem, namely, extra pay for work on these holidays.	1. Were the arguments of the M.C. marshalled in good order ? 2. Did it appear that he was prepared ? 3. What was his purpose in introducing item 14 ? 4. Was he giving emps. an alternative ? 5. Was this a good time to suggest alternatives ? 6. Was it sound procedure to weight the "responsibility to the public" arguments ? 7. Were his arguments of the kind likely to open or close discussion ? 8. Were his arguments logically sound ?

a	b	c
Sequence of events in the Committee session as derived from the record.	*The Chairman's conduct as derived from interpretations of the record.*	*Conference procedure questions to be used by research agents in a group interview with the chairman of the committee, the participant observer, and several other Management officials involved in committee operations.*
IV.—continued 13. But it is understood that you are not interested in this phase of the problem, but merely in getting the holidays. 14. We want uniformity as far as it is possible; we do not wish to play favourites. 15. But, so long as the traffic force is on the job, the major part of our installation and practically all of our maintenance forces must be on duty. 16. Therefore we feel we have no good grounds to ask for the extension of holidays privileges.		
V. At this point the M.C. asked: 1. If there were remaining points not covered; 2. If the group wished to express itself.	1. He was again " putting it up to the group." 2. He appeared to wish to include all possible factors.	1. Were the questions of the M.C. put for the purpose of: (a) Rounding out the arguments? (b) Securing assent to his position? (c) Precipitating discussion?

The above illustrative material, if carried out completely, would obviously be too bulky for publication and, furthermore, nothing new as illustration of the technique under discussion would be added. Consequently it is terminated at this point.

III. *Corrective points of reference derived from the participant observers and other participants in the meeting.*

With the presentation of the above analysis and interpretation of the research agents to the group a discussion followed based upon the questions contained therein. The chairman was asked if he thought that the real issue was the question of holidays. He thought that it was, but added that he expected the case to be reopened as a wage issue some time later, that is, in the form of a request for overtime pay on holidays. Since the employees had presented a request to a management chairman in advance of the meeting, he, as representative of the management, was prepared with an answer. It appeared then that from the standpoint of the research agent's analysis of the meeting the management chairman was limited as to what he could do since the management had decided not to comply with the request for additional holidays. His function then was to defend management, and he therefore could not allow the issue to be opened.

In explaining his preliminary remarks to the group, the management chairman said that he considered the employee chairman's statement of the case as a criticism of management policy. Consequently he felt obliged to defend and justify management.

It appeared further that when at point V (in preceding analysis) he, as chairman, put the matter up to the group, he was not opening up the question of holidays, but rather he was asking for a consensus on his statement of management's position.

In this manner the research agents gained an insight

into some of the motives underlying the strictly verbal report of the account which they had received.

According to the participant observer's account of the meeting, he said that all the employee representatives had taken part in the discussion, but that only the management chairman and one other management representative had taken part. The participant observer thought that the mood and tempo of this discussion were even and regular throughout. No anger or intense feeling had been observable. Apparently the chairman, in officiating, had performed the following functions :

(a) He supplied facts.
(b) He interpreted policies and principles.
(c) He justified management by meeting criticism.
(d) He refined, delimited and localized the issue.
(e) He made various discriminations.

Participant Observing as a Specialized Tool.

Analysis of the above record and interpretation of participant observation indicates that this technique reveals many general facts concerning committees and their process. As used in this study, participant observing was directed, however, toward two special aspects, namely, the chairman's conduct and conference procedure. The record provides a clear picture of the chairman's rôle and the manner in which this influences the total committee process. It will be seen, for example, how the chairman's early announcement of his attitude toward the solution of the problem set the tone for ensuing discussion ; once the participants were aware that the chairman had " made up his mind " they realized that the remainder of the discussion would be one in which " side-taking " and matching of force would be the principal elements. Consequently, the tone of the conference was one of " bloc " and " defeat ", with a remote opportunity for compromise. With this sort of picture of committee process available, the research agents, and readers as well, may construct a fairly accurate interpretation of the chairman's personality, his conception of his rôle as chairman, and the quality of conference procedure which these factors would allow.

The theory of participant observing is relatively simple and in unorganized form is in general use, especially by those who wish to control social processes. Its application is, however, exceedingly difficult and complex. The above presentation omits more than it includes, and in the interest of those who may wish to experiment further with this technique we suggest a sample list of questions asked of a participant observer.

Types of Questions Asked of the Participant Observer by the Research Agents :

A. *The given situation :*

(*a*) Is there anything significant about this particular conference ?

(*b*) What has happened in previous meetings of this group which may have some bearing upon the present session ?

(*c*) Are there any new elements present ?

B. *The rôle of the chairman :*

(*a*) Does the chairman use an agenda ?

(*b*) Does the agenda appear to patternize the group's response ?

(c) Does the chairman act as though he were fully aware of the specialized function he performs ?

(d) Does he keep before the group a total view of the problem under discussion ?

(e) Does he defend or espouse his or someone else's views ?

(f) Does he put questions in such form as to elicit prompt and willing responses ?

(g) Does he at times appear to dominate the group ?

(h) Does he appear to place a different weight upon the contributions of different members of the group ?

(i) Does he ever close discussion arbitrarily ?

(j) Is he skilful in revealing the " hot spots " in the discussion ?

(k) Does he make sure that all views and interests are expressed ?

(l) Does he clarify issues in his re-statements and summaries ?

(m) Does he seem to be aware of certain tensions between members ?

(n) Is he skilful at drawing out the backward members ?

C. *Personality differences :*

(a) Are the management representatives uniform in type ?

(b) Are the employee representatives uniform in type ?

(c) What are the chief traits of each group ?

(d) Are there any outstanding personalities in either group ?

(e) Do the employees generally depend upon one or two persons to represent their views ? Who are these persons ?

(f) Does the management group likewise depend upon one or two to represent its views, and who ?

(g) Are there any sharp personality differences which lead to tensions, inhibitions, misunderstandings ?

D. *Quantity and quality of participation :*

(a) Is participation general ?

(b) Who does most talking ?

(c) Does amount of participation vary with the subject ?

(d) Does initiator talk more when his subject is under discussion ?

(e) What proportion of the total participation is made by

    i. the management chairman ;

    ii. the employee chairman ?

(f) Is there a tendency to participate in general or in specific terms ?

(g) Are facts contributed ?

(h) Experience ?

(i) At what points does participation seem to lag ?

E. *The rôle of the representative :*

   (*a*) Do representatives speak as if they were representing ?

   (*b*) Are there spokesmen for each side who seem to do most of the representing ?

   (*c*) Does the group look to certain representatives for specialized contributions ?

   (*d*) Are there any " loud-speaker " representatives?

   (*e*) By what signs is it known that the representative speaks for his group, or for himself ?

   (*f*) What fraction of the worker's personality gets represented predominantly ?

F. *Characteristic reactions and interactions :*

   (*a*) Do various representatives appear to react to each other positively ? Negatively ?

   (*b*) Is there a marked difference between the interactions between representatives, and between representatives and the chairman ?

   (*c*) Are there any members of the group toward whom the reactions of representatives are habitually in terms of authority ?

   (*d*) Are there interactions in which the habitual mood is one of humour, or fun-making ?

   (*e*) What interactions appear to lead the group forward toward constructive action ?

   (*f*) What interactions appear to impede the group's progress ?

   (*g*) Do interactions change when the matter under discussion obviously reveals interest-distance?

G. *Cycles of tempo and tone :*

(a) Does discussion proceed slowly and haltingly at first ?

(b) Is good-fellowship manifest at the beginning ?

(c) Is there present an obvious mood of expectancy ?

(d) Is there present an obvious mood of non-expectancy ?

(e) At what points do moods change ?

(f) Is participation more general and lively at given points ?

(g) Is indifference apparent at given points ?

(h) At what points does attention rise and fall ?

(i) Are there obvious resistances and tensions ?

(j) Is it apparent that there are present certain overtones or undertones which prevent frankness and impede discussion ?

(k) Does the mood of attention and interest heighten when a given case comes to the stage of conclusion ?

(l) When voting is utilized, is the response animated or listless ?

(m) Do participants approach problems by roundabout, or direct paths ? Does this vary ?

(n) What mood is evident when long speeches are made ?

(o) Is it ever apparent that the conclusion reached is disapproved although not openly ?

(p) What happens when the meeting is over ? Do participants appear to be eager to go on discussing certain questions ? Has good fellowship increased or diminished ?

L

CHAPTER XI

(Basic Form : The Person-to-Event Relationship)

" THE definition of an event by assignment of demarcations," states Whitehead,[1] " is an arbitrary act of thought corresponding to no perceptual experience. Thus it is a basal assumption essential for ratiocination relating to perceptual experience that there are definite entities which are events." Professor Whitehead appears to make three affirmations in the above statement, namely (a) that the flow of experience does not of itself reveal definite demarcations which may be called events ; (b) that this assignment of demarcations is an arbitrary act of thought, and (c) that such an arbitrary assignment of demarcations, denoting entities, is essential as an assumption if events are to become a part of perceptual experience. Simple as these statements may appear, they constitute one of the most critical problems for scientific method. Each separate science must continue to ask : *What is an event ?* In the physical sciences events are assumed to be forces as related to objects ; thus a change in the position of an object constitutes an event. The physicist may assign demarcations to an event of this sort by measurements of mass, density, volume, motion, acceleration, expansion, direction, et cetera. In the process of measuring, his basic assumptions concerning the event and his perceptual experience as related to the event,

[1] A. N. Whitehead : *The Principle of Natural Knowledge.*

appear to drop from the equation. In the social sciences arbitrariness of demarcation is greater and measuring techniques are less developed ; consequently, social events are usually described in such naïve terms as to make the description valueless, or are merely the personal imposition of an individual observer.

Our present concern is with a limited class of events, those which go by the name of " events of human association, communication and participation," to use the language of Professor Dewey.[1] Such events are essentially psychic and cannot, therefore, be adequately described until more reliable psychological tools of analysis are available. Lacking some of these tools, social research is obliged to make even more bold and arbitrary demarcations of events than is true of some of the other sciences. From a psycho-sociological point of view an event may be thought of as a change in the relational aspects of social units. The event itself is an interruption of habit-experience, consciously recognized as such by the participants, or arbitrarily demarcated as such by an observer. Thus, social experience may be said to flow as a line more or less straight, without *eventful*ness.

(a) ———————————————————————————————

or, it may be said to flow in undulations with nodes and internodes :

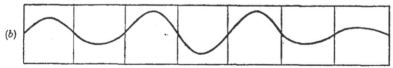

(b)

---

[1] *Experience and Nature*, Chapter VII. In this volume Professor Dewey suggests a classification of events consisting of physical, psycho-physical, and mental.

The vertical lines in the above graph of experience represent arbitrary demarcations of events ; the social scientist, then, observes particularly what transpires within the margins of two arbitrary lines inserted by himself at given points in the flow of experience.

Experience within an industry consists of continuing communications and participations, and the entire flow of this experience may be thought of as a sequence of events. A formal meeting of employees and managers constitutes an event which may be more readily demarcated, set off from the general flow of experience because the participants themselves regard such a meeting as something different from the usual flow of experience. As research agents our task with respect to events of this character was to conduct such experiments as might reveal to the observer something of the quality of communication and participation within the setting of a joint committee session. The major event, therefore, is the total committee session ; within this event are subsidiary events which, if susceptible of observation, should reveal knowledge with respect to the quality of interaction which characterizes the behaviour of employees and managers when acting as members of a joint committee.

At first glance it might appear that such observation could be accomplished most effectively if verbatim records of the proceedings were taken, either by a stenographer or a dictaphone. Each item of participation in the total flow of communication would thus be made available to the observers. But, communication is not simply a process of verbalization. Indeed, the spoken word is frequently unimportant in communication, save as related with tone, gesture, bodily position, et cetera. The observer will, obviously, pay special attention to verbal communications since these will constitute his main resource for deriving logical meanings, but he will also attend to the non-verbal accompaniments of communication, its undertones and overtones, which in the end will make his meanings psychological as well as logical. Civilized people do, of course, tend to become word-conscious; they attempt to express all meanings in terms of words. But, to neglect the physiological substratum is to make of communication a wholly rational affair, a procedure which in the end falsifies our interpretations of behaviour.[1]

Technical methods for observing communication as verbal (symbolical), and as non-verbal (physiological), are still wanting. The chief difficulty lies in the fact that communication itself proceeds in wholes, not parts: the spoken word and the lifted arm, the threatening gesture, or the increased volume of tone happen as one, not two units of behaviour. When the observer separates the word from the gesture he is simply being arbitrary in analysis. The second difficulty resides in the fact that the observer, whether he wishes it or not, will " see what he is looking for." Observation is not a direct response of the eye, or ear, or hand, but is based upon the response of a great mass of previous habits, bodily responses, movements, et cetera. " We observe with our whole past

---

[1] Dr. Trigant Burrow, a psychoanalyst, appears to believe that this separation of the symbolical from the biological represents an actual danger to mental health. See " Social Images versus Reality," *The Journal of Abnormal and Social Psychology*, 1924, XIX, 230.

of psychological experience."[1]   Observation, implicitly, is a selective procedure; what appears to be meaningful to any given observer is so because of his past experience, plus his perceptual capacities.[2] Naïve observation cannot, patently, be accepted as a trustworthy technique for social research.

With these two major difficulties in mind, we may now proceed to describe the techniques of observation which have been utilized in this study. Our aim was to reveal the dynamics of committee process, utilizing direct observation of events as a technique which might illuminate certain aspects of process more fully than other techniques. Before direct observations began we had already familiarized ourselves with such general information as the range of subjects dealt with by such committees, the general conceptions of conference method in vogue, et cetera, and consequently, it was possible to minimize certain items, or at least, to reduce them to lower levels of attention. In terms of committee dynamics we aimed particularly to secure information of the following variety :

(1) *Time :*

(*a*) Time consumed by the total meeting ;

(*b*) Time consumed in discussing specific items.

(2) *Subject-matter :*

(a) Simple denotation of the subject or subjects dealt with at a given committee session.

(3) *Participation :*

(*a*) Range of participation ;   ⎰ See Chapter
(*b*) The mode of participation.   ⎱ on Charting.

---

[1] J. F. Markey, Chapter III, *Trends in American Sociology.*
[2] See Chapter III, *Gestalt Psychology,* by W. Köhler.

(4) *Overt, non-verbal behaviour :*
(a) Tone of voice, gestures, facial expressions, et cetera, accompanying communication.

(5) *Conference procedure :*
(a) The generalized framework of conference within which the communication and participation takes place. (See Chapter V.)

(6) *Chairman's conduct :*
(a) Range of his participation ;
(b) Impositions of procedure emanating from him ;
(c) His special objects of attention.

(7) *Tempo of Interaction :*
(a) Speed of communication.

(8) *Treatment of Difference :*
(a) Differences on points of fact ;
(b) On points of opinion ;
(c) Differences apparent but unexpressed.

(9) *Conclusions reached :*
(a) How items of business are disposed of ;
(b) General tone of group at the point of decision.

Utilizing the above suggested points of observation, the following chart gives a tabular arrangement of the facts in a particular meeting showing the distribution of time, the subjects discussed, the procedure of the meeting from the point of view of the chairman and the representatives. The third column gives the observer's interpretative comment based upon the particularized points of reference discussed above. The last column shows how the committee procedure and the interpretative analysis throw light upon the categories, Impulsion, Circumjacence, Interaction and Emergence.

OBSERVATION OF COMMITTEE

Time	Procedure		Interpretative Comment	Reference to Categories
	Management Chairman	Group		
11 : 03	M.C. introduces visitor. M.C. tells of his experience re nomination of two employees who wished later to withdraw.	Dialogue and exchange of information with M.C.	The chairman's manner is informal.	*Circumjacence :* Mgt. and Emp. attitudes revealed.
11 : 10	The minutes of the previous meeting are distributed and read.	There is exchange of comment bet. M.C. and E. Reps.	The subject-matter seems secondary to the reassuring tone of discourse.	*Circumjacence :* Mgt. and Emp. attitudes revealed.
11 : 17	M.C. opens discussion by asking "What have you on your minds?" M.C. restates case for clarification and this is followed by exchange bet. E.R.'s and M.C. M.C. puts matter on personal basis of confidence and agrees to take up problem at Superintendent's meeting.	E.R. responds by stating difficulty in arrangements for punching time-clock at lunch.	Tone of meeting is that of frank and open discussion, very informal and friendly. The M.C. is skilful in drawing out the employees.	*Circumjacence :* Mgt. pattern of dealing with cases is suggested by chairman's disposition. *Interaction :* Emp. response to M.C. indicates lack of inhibiting factor.

OBSERVATION OF COMMITTEE—*continued*

Time	Procedure		Interpretative Comment	Reference to Categories
	Management Chairman	Group		
11 : 25	M.C. to second member, " What do you think ? " M.C. draws out member to clarify case. M.C. agrees to investigate case.	E.R. complains about truck having broken sidewalk and drain, causing flooded area.	The prevailing tone of the meeting continues.	
11 : 30	 M.C. replies that as long as everybody is satisfied things are all right. M.C. explains company action in this case. He seeks assurance of the company's action.	E.R. reports improvement in method of wage payment. Member gives history of grievance on method of payment which he had settled previously	The atmosphere is apparently genuine. Reps. seem to be at ease. General positive comment by M.C. and E.R.'s	*Interaction :* Exchange facilitated by pleasant recollection of previous experience.
11 : 36	M.C. " Jimmie, what have you on your mind ? "	E.R. has nothing to report. He comments on the moving of a piece of machinery.	At this time the tone of the meeting is lowered due to a lag in responses. Chairman has made rounds asking each E.R. for any complaints he might have.	

OBSERVATION OF COMMITTEE—*continued*

Time	Procedure		Interpretative Comment	Reference to Categories
	Management Chairman	Group		
11 : 38	M.C. is conciliatory ; he draws out E.R. on basis of complaint by using specific question. M.C. agrees to take up matter.	E.R. complains about the houseman of a company official and his interference with the men. E.R. reiterates.	This complaint is probably semi-personal, but it seems to come out because there is no pressure for time or action.	*Circumjacence :* Informal nature of procedure induces men to speak out.
11 : 48	M.C. initiates discussion amount of full-time work during the past year. He explains new policy of Co. in working out programme in advance to smooth out working curve.		M.C. talks personally and directly to the men. His manner is persuasive and convincing as he assures employees of company's motives.	*Impulsion :* Mgt.'s purpose to keep emps. aware of Mgt. policy.
11 : 50	M.C. gives figures and data on policy of maintenance dept.	E.R. comments on improvement in working time arrangement. He asks questions about a certain roof. Would replacement sooner be better than constant repair?	The meeting is unwinding as time for adjournment approaches.	

The Observation Sheet.

For extensive observation using the maximum number of points of reference the research agent must have an unobstructed view of the meeting place and of all the participants. This latter is only possible when the group is limited in number, that is, preferably not more than fifteen. A columnal arrangement of the categories of observation will facilitate speed in recording and symbols for the units of participation may be used as suggested in the chapter on charting. In this way, the purpose of the observation chart, to show a summarized picture of important aspects of committee process is achieved. In circumstances where extensive note-taking is not advisable, the observer can record three important aspects of the conference in the following way :

Time	Event Progress of discussion	Process Comment
10 : 00 10 : 06		

By the aid of his wrist-watch the observer can at frequent intervals note the time. This will give a distribution of the subject or subjects discussed throughout the meeting. Under the heading Event, he can note the subject-matter and its ramifications, and in the last column his value comments.

CHAPTER XII

THE TECHNIQUE OF CASE ANALYSIS

(*Basic Form : The Person-to-Record Relationship*)

MOST of the stereotyped business of joint committees is unimportant, being nothing more than the routine characteristic of any organized group. These ordinary and routinized affairs of committees are, however, worth noting since they furnish indices of habits and customs. But, what an investigator really wishes to know about an organized group is the manner of its functioning when confronted with situations which call for choices, decisions. Events of this nature tend to become the nodal points by which the activities of the group are recollected and recorded ; such records attain increasing importance since they become incorporated in the control tradition of the group. It is these events which describe the quality of the social process, and when they leave their traces in permanent records they constitute one of the major data-sources for research.[1]

A record is " a mark or trace that serves as a memorial giving enduring attestation of an event or fact,"[2] and certain historical sciences, notably anthropology, archæology and palæontology utilize such sources almost

---

[1] Certain so-called " objectivists " confine themselves entirely to such sources of fact, believing that persons and events themselves are unreliable for research purposes. See *Methods and Status of Scientific Research*, by Spahr and Swenson.

[2] Standard Dictionary.

exclusively. The social sciences (sociology, economics, political science, and history), being primarily concerned with events occurring in the more recent past, or contemporaneously, have occasion to use the more common form of record, namely, the written word. There is still considerable dispute with respect to the highest scientific use which may be made of written accounts of events. The historians, for example, continue their perennial debate concerning which events should be included and which excluded, and more important still, the manner of selecting, interpreting and validifying the written records upon which their researches are based.

There are at least two technical approaches to written records used as social data, namely : (*a*) Selection of separate categories within the records and reduction of these to statistical terms ; (*b*) isolation of given contextual sequences in events for purpose of detailed analysis according to the technique which is usually called " case study." We have experimented with both of the foregoing techniques in the present study, and this chapter is concerned with the latter.

Defining Case Analysis.

The following terms frequently are used indiscriminately and must therefore be distinguished : *case study, case method, case record, case history.* Approximate definitions will suffice for present purposes :

Case Study : The analysis of an abstracted phase of experience, usually performed in the interest of describing some quality in the experiential whole.

Case Method : A term utilized primarily in applied sociology and implying that diagnostic and therapeutic approaches to the solution of a problem may be made by considering the involved situation as unique and discrete. Case method is also used in connection with teaching, *e.g.*, the case method of teaching law and social work, the connotation being that the student learns facts and principles through the analysis of relevant case histories.

Case Record : The formal or informal statement of a case set forth verbally or symbolically.

Case History : A case record arranged in chronological sequence.

The process, then, of abstracting some phase of experience is one which has been found useful in social diagnostics, therapeutics, teaching, and history. In what sense is such a procedure useful also to social research ?

" Case study method," writes Shaw, " emphasizes the total situation or combination of factors, the description of the process or sequence of events in which behaviour occurs, the study of individual behaviour in its total setting, and the analysis and comparison of cases leading to formulation of hypotheses."[1] Case studies, then, are to furnish a total view, " to take into account the richness of fact "[2] concerning human events. We now see why the case study method (technique) has become so popular

---

[1] " Case Study Method," by C. R. Shaw : *Publications of the American Sociological Society*, Vol. 21, p. 149.

[2] " The Contributions of Case Studies to Sociology," by W. Healy, *Publications of the American Sociological Society*, Vol. 18, p. 154.

during the past two or three decades : Scientists and philosophers have during this period criticized the so-called "atomistic" conception of research ; they, the critics, have insisted that the reduction of reality to smaller and smaller units would not in the end lead to more important fact or truth. On the contrary, so the critics contended, " atomism " represents a limited point of view, both for science and philosophy. What is needed in order to give these ever-smaller units of reality meaning is a view of the total situation within which they operate. *Gestalt Psychology* [1] may be regarded as a direct result of the revolt against " atomism," and case analysis is its counterpart in the social sciences.

The Partially-total Situation.

The term " total situation " is obviously too broad for any technique of research. No technique or combination of techniques capable of revealing the totality of any event is as yet in existence. Case studies, it might preferably be said, aim to supplement the kind of facts which are revealed by subdivision of units through the process of viewing these same facts in a larger context. This approach to the study of phenomena is, patently, arbitrary ; in the first place, the observer selects out of some comprehensive totality some item which seems to him significant ; he then utilizes whatever records are available, again a selective procedure, and thereafter supplements the records with answers to queries formulated by himself, once more a selective procedure. What is finally described as a result of case analysis is a partially-total

[1] See particularly the writings of Koffka and Köhler.

situation, limited by the available records and the observer's various gradients of perception.

The Categories of Case Analysis.

Considerable attention is now being directed toward refining case analysis as a technique for social research. A monograph entitled *Case Study Possibilities*,[1] is probably the best single piece of work in this area. This monograph suggests a procedure for deriving inductive categories for case analysis and then suggests the following terms :

(*a*) The Fact Items : the heterogeneous fact items as collected in the case records ;

(*b*) The Social Facts : fact items as belonging to minor clusters ;

(*c*) The Social Fact Groups : groups of minor clusters arranged to show wider relatedness ;

(*d*) The Type of Case : inspection of the social fact groups indicates the general title for the case.[2]

It will be seen that the derivation of the above categories involves deductive as well as inductive elements. To impute importance to anything is in itself a deductive procedure. This is not, from our point of view, a hindrance to research since we have all along admitted that human purpose enters into and gives colour to all research.

---

[1] By Ada Sheffield.

[2] Groupings of the (*c*) variety, and designation of the type case should, according to Mrs. Sheffield, flow from social import as imputed by the observer. " Social meaning, therefore, is a property, not of single fact items as a rule, but of a group of items, interpretation and its descriptive terms should be applied to the smallest group of fact items which has a social import " (p. 54).

A natural classification such as the one suggested above results, however, in one thing, a name for the case. What is needed in Case Analysis is a set of significant categories for the analysis of these aggregated fact items. But significant facts are purposive facts and until this purpose is stated no such set of categories is possible.

In the present study the purpose is the analysis of joint committee procedure, problem and result. Case study categories therefore must derive from this purpose.

Case Analysis then, consists of three major steps, namely :

(1) The apprehending, discovering, and amassing of facts ;

(2) The analysis of these facts by various kinds of discrimination ;

(3) The interpretation of these facts, including imputation of values.

Considered in the light of the joint committee in industry, and as used in the present study, these three steps may be further elaborated :

(1) *The facts* to be utilized in case study method are of three varieties :

(a) Facts which constitute the essence of the case ; facts within the industrial setting and the relations between employees and management.

(b) Facts which emerge as the case is discussed or dealt with by various committees of individuals.

(c) Facts which are descriptive of the effect upon the case caused by its treatment by groups and individuals.

M

(The given data, the derived data, and the precipitated data. Given in the case; derived from discussion of the case and impinged upon the case by the representative process.)

(2) *Analysis* includes the following kinds of discriminations:

(*a*) Discriminations between various kinds of groups.

(*b*) Discriminations between various kinds of facts.

(*c*) Discriminations between various kinds of authoritative individuals.

(*d*) Discriminations between various kinds of group processes.

(*e*) Discriminations between various kinds of conclusions.

(3) *Interpretation* may consist of the following ways of ascribing values:

(*a*) Values derived from the powers of the groups.

(*b*) Values derived from the participant character of the representatives.

(*c*) Values derived from the method of conference used.

(*d*) Values derived from the method of securing and utilizing emergent facts.

(*e*) Values derived from the nature of the conclusion.

A Proposed Form for Recording Case Materials.

Assuming that all the data constituting a case are in hand, it then becomes necessary to relate this material to the total research purpose. What is this material expected to reveal ? In order to reduce all case data to comparable terms we are suggesting a form, not usable for all case studies of course, but one which was found suitable for the study of joint committees :

I. *Factual :*

　1. Chronology of dates of significant events in development of case.

II. *Conference Progression :*

　1. The nature of the problem.
　　(*a*) How is the problem recognized ?
　　(*b*) Is the question defined ?
　　(*c*) Ramifications or delimitations of the question.

　2. Interest distance in the issue.
　　(*a*) Background factors giving emotional depth.
　　(*b*) Particular points of emotional strain.

　3. At what point is the validity of the factual basis of the discussion questioned ?
　　(*a*) What differences are there on matters of fact ?
　　(*b*) What differences are there on matters of opinion ?
　　(*c*) When are principal facts brought in ?

　4. What explorations of differences of fact and what discussion of differences of opinion ?
　　(*a*) What are the data on differences as to fact ?
　　(*b*) What can be said as to differences as to point of view ?

　5. The kinds of conference method employed at different stages.

III. *What are the Possible Courses of Action ?*

    (*a*) Analysis of the factors in II. above with con-figurated statement of the whole case.

    (*b*) What is or was actual course of action ?

IV. *The Conclusion Reached Varied in Terms of these Suggested Values :*

    (*a*) Conference method that leads to constructive solutions ?

    (*b*) Educational growth and development for the participants ?

    (*c*) Greater effectiveness of the conference as a step in the industrial process ?

    (*d*) Social ramifications of the joint experience.

A Sample Case Analysed.

The following summarized presentation is divided into three major parts, namely (*a*) Chronology, (*b*) Interpretation, and (*c*) Interpretation in terms of the four categories of research, namely, Impulsion, Circumjacence, Interaction, and Emergence. In this case we have followed through, by the use of records, a case involving both committee and extra-committee activities. The employees initiated the case by asking for a change in holiday schedule. From this point onward the reader may review the case as it evolves through numerous processes and stages.

Chronology	Interpretation	Interpretation in terms of Categories
1. Gen. Mgr. refers to wish of employees for change in holiday work schedule. (To be off night of holiday rather than night before.)	Question apparently arose outside of committee and was brought in by Mgt. Chairman	*Impulsion :* Employee desire to change established schedule. *Circumjacence:* Evidence of contact of Emp. Rep. and Mgt. Chair. outside of committee meeting.
2. Emp. Reps. meeting separately vote for change to night of holiday.	Situation carried forward by employee vote.	*Impulsion :* Employees carry matter further.
3. Mgt. Chr. agrees to take up matter as decided by emps.		*Interaction :* Response takes place in meeting following vote.
4. Exchange of letters Mgt. to Mgt. (1) explaining case, (2) replying that company thought change inadvisable.	Mgt. decision from outside committee against employée request.	*Circumjacence :* Apparently it is the custom to make such decisions in this manner.
5. Employees' committee voice regret at not having answer from Mgt.	Interest-distance indicated. A holiday has come and Mgt. has not answered.	*Impulsion :* (Repulsion).
6. Mgt. advises Mgt. Chairman that negative answer was to be considered " unofficial."	" Unofficial " apparently meant that since the matter had been lifted from the committee by the Mgt. Chairman the case could now await further employee action by formal use of the committee.	*Circumjacence :* Apparently there is a double understanding of procedure.
7. Employees continue discussion indicating regret at Mgt. position as well as misunderstanding of status of the case. Final appeal to Federal authority suggested.	Interest-distance widening. Employee hostility evoked.	*Impulsion:* (Repulsion) Employees' antipathy to Mgt. voiced.
8. Mgt. to Mgt. memo. referring to employee proposal to take question to Federal authority as allowed in plan.		

Chronology	Interpretation	Interpretation in terms of Categories
9. At annual conference of all emp. reps. and Mgt., Pres. of company thought change could be made. Vice-Pres. says privately that he thought matter could be straightened out.	Situation enlarged by discussion of problem in wider setting of corporation policy.	*Interaction :* Consideration of subject has now reached highest company authority and in most significant committee setting. *Circumjacence :* Procedure of cases indicated by having important Co. officials' evidence consideration at employee request.
10. Emp. Chairman reports to Emp. committee about his conversations with Gen. Mgr. that there is no answer from the " higher up " mgt. authority with whom the case is resting.	The emp. chair. is apparently carrying on discussion about the case outside of the committee.	*Circumjacence :* Apparently there are all kinds of informal modes of extra committee procedure.
11. Emps. request information as to status of case. Emp. Chr. reports no definite answer.	They can only await whatever Mgt. decision is reached.	*Impulsion :* Employee persistence indicated.
12. Employees again request information from Emp. Chr. as to status of case. He replies that Gen. Mgr. reports no answer from corporation headquarters.	Another holiday has come and men are uncertain as to working schedules. Regret that highest corporation officials have not kept promise.	*Impulsion :* (Repulsion).
13. Gen. Mgr. reports to employee representatives that he has taken up matter with corporation officials, asking for a conclusion, and received assurance that it would be taken care of.	Since it is a large corporation with many plants the problem is not merely a local one but has to be viewed in terms of the whole corporation and its policies.	*Circumjacence :* Since the matter is not to be decided by the local mgt. the local mgt. is really a third party.
14. Gen. Mgr. reports to employee committee that matter has been decided according to their original request.	Conclusion is reached by corporation officials and reported to local company and then passed on to the employees.	*Circumjacence :* Concluding step in handling problem indicating management's conception of procedure.

CHAPTER XIII

THE TECHNIQUE OF CHARTING

(*Basic Form : The Person-to-Record Relationship.*)

CASE analysis is a technique which may be, and usually is, employed for the purpose of clarifying historical data. The basic material of a case is a description of an event which has occurred so far in the past as to allow for isolation, delimitation, and abstraction. In most instances the person who analyses the case material is not the same person who has had first-hand contact with the event ; consequently, the analyser is compelled to construct meanings and interpretations which are, essentially, thrice removed from reality. Analysis of this sort is, obviously, subject to the vagaries of individual gradients, since no two persons are likely to arrive at the same conception of meanings from the given data of any specific case. This liability of historical case analysis has led to the wish for techniques which might come nearer the current event. Social scientists, as well as all other scientists, are eager to discover ways of analysing the living present, the fleeting event which can never be reconstructed with fidelity once memory is called upon to intervene.

Thus, in the study of joint committees we have wished to come closer to the actual events of a committee session than is possible by the use of historical records. We have already described how far direct and participant observation carries us in this direction. Another possibility was recognized, namely, the transference of the event to graphic forms [1] as quickly as possible after the committee session. In order to test this technique it became necessary to secure verbatim records of committee meetings ; these records were then reduced to units of communication, and both the units and the lines of communication were indicated upon a chart. The reader may then follow the progressing line of communication as it flows from one person to another in the group, and thus see at a glance some of the relationships between the problem under discussion and the method of conference in use.

What is the Unit of Participation ?

A unit of participation consists of a remark or expression which in its primary meaning reveals that the speaker is attempting to (*a*) make a statement, or (*b*) ask a question. In each case, the statement or the question may be either relevant or irrelevant to the subject under discussion. Statements, in addition to their relevancy or irrelevancy, may be classified according to their main purport or most obvious intention ; thus it is found that some statements are made in order to introduce facts into the discussion, others are plainly argumentative and still others have to do with the conference proceeding itself.   Questions,

[1] " Simple data, as well as those that do not yield readily to such methods of analysis, may also require careful reshuffling or reworking in order to exhaust the various points of view from which these data may be studied. No possibility of manipulation should be overlooked which may lead to suggestions of meanings and ideas, or to the accurate testing of different hypotheses. . . . Their great value (graphs) lies in their appeal to the visual sense and in the high degree of clarity with which relationships may be brought out."—*How to do Research Work*, by W. C. Schluter.

likewise, may be classified according to their main purport, and thus it will be found that questions are asked (*a*) for the purpose of securing actual information, (*b*) for the purpose of revealing opinion, (*c*) for the purpose of securing a clearer understanding of a previous statement, or (*d*) for the purpose of eliciting experience from others.

The above varieties of statements (factual, argumentative, procedural) may be still further refined in terms of specific implications. For example, a statement may be made in the form of a report, it may be merely a straightforward fact, an item of experience, a reference to the constitution or by-laws or to rules, an announcement, or a comparison. This process of refining the classifications may, of course, be carried to such limits as to make the categories useless for analysis. In order to keep the categories representative of units of participation within manageable terms it seems advisable to adhere to the smallest possible number, keeping in mind, however, the necessity of conveying a realistic picture of what actually takes place in a committee session. With this delimiting principle in mind, we propose to utilize the following categories as symbols for varying units of participation :

I. Statements which are either relevant or irrelevant and

   A. Factual :
       1. Purporting to present a report :
           (*a*) based upon investigation ;
           (*b*) transmitted from another committee ;
           (*c*) secured from an authority.

2. Purporting to express a general fact :
3. Purporting to relate an experience :
4. Purporting to announce a changed policy, practice, rule, et cetera :
5. Purporting to draw a comparison.

B. Argumentative :

1. Purporting to express an opinion :
2. Purporting to rebut a previous statement :
3. Purporting to offer a suggestion for consideration :
4. Purporting to interpret a meaning :
5. Purporting to challenge or contend :
6. Purporting to reveal agreement :
7. Purporting to admonish.

C. Procedural :

1. Purporting to remind members of an item on rules of procedure, rules of order, constitution, et cetera :
2. Purporting to announce some fact of procedure :
3. Purporting to modify or alter procedure.

II. Questions which are either relevant or irrelevant and

A. Are asked for the purpose of securing information :

B. Are asked for the purpose of securing an opinion :

C. Are asked for the purpose of clarifying understanding of a statement, decision, et cetera :

D. Are asked for the purpose of securing statements
of experience from others.[1]

Substituting initials and numerals as symbols for the
above units of participation for charting purposes, we
may designate a relevant statement, factual, and purporting to give a report as: R S F—1. Thenceforth
all factual statements would be differentiated by one of
the remaining numerals in the series under Factual.
An item representing a relevant statement, argumentative, purporting to reveal an opinion would be designated: R S A—1, and thus onward with this series.
A unit representing an irrelevant statement would be
denoted simply as I S F, or I S A; in case the apparently irrelevant statement proved later to have a
definite relationship to the subject under discussion,
this fact would be noted by the addition of a numeral
indicating its main purport, thus such a statement
indicating that the purport had been to relate an experience would be designated: I S F—3. Relevant
questions may be symbolized similarly; thus, a relevant
question calling for information would be indicated as
R Q—inf.; for an opinion R Q—op.; for clarification
R Q—cl.; and for experience R Q—ex. In case the
query appears to have greater import than any of these
four classifications imply, a numeral may be selected from
the sub-classification of statements, thus indicating an

[1] In the case of an irrelevant question it is not necessary to designate
the purport. If, however, subsequent analysis reveals that what
seemed irrelevant at the moment turns out to be definitely related, a
proper denotation needs to be made. In most instances, however,
irrelevant statements and questions are purely rhetorical, proceed
from inattention, lack of knowledge, or the felt need for release.

affinity of purport.   Thus, if one wished to indicate that a question was not merely relevant, and not merely for purposes of securing information, but was specifically related to a report, the symbol might be R Q in.—1.

In order to add further meaning to the chart some indication should be given with respect to the amount of time devoted to each unit of participation.   The above symbols used in a chart would indicate the distribution plus the type of participation in the discussion.   Longitudinal spacing on the chart would, in turn, indicate the relative amount of time consumed by each unit of participation.   Since the units of participation have been found to be almost uniform in length, we have allowed only a single longitudinal space for each unit ; when one person combines more than one unit in his discourse, the units are tabulated in order and thus the chart readily reveals the relative amount of time taken in discussion by any one person.   Before proceeding with further analysis of the symbols utilized it may be advisable to furnish a sample chart.   (See opposite page.)

Interpreting the Graphic Analysis.

Mere presentation of what took place in a committee meeting is the first step in analysis.   The symbolization and placement of units of participation provides a picture of interaction within a committee setting.   The meaning of this interaction in terms of conference procedure must now be deduced by further steps in analysis.   Reference to this chart will indicate two additional phases of analysis which are tentatively proposed.

Units of participation tend to group themselves about

ANALYSIS AND INTERPRETATION OF JOINT COMMITTEE PROCEDURE

The chart consists of two major divisions, namely Analysis and Interpretation. Under Analysis, Column (*a*) indicates each successive unit of participation. Column (*b*) indicates the Management Representatives consisting of four plus the Management Chairman who presides. Column (*c*) indicates the Employee Representatives consisting of eight plus a chairman and two visitors. The heavy line running from the square of one person to the square of another indicates the flow of participation. Column (*d*) consists of methodology interpretations of various phases or periods of the conference procedure, and Column (*e*) comprises some psychological interpretations mainly of dominant attitudes.

separate phases or periods in a discussion procedure. The various meanings which we have ascribed to such groupings will be found under the heading "Methodological." It appeared, for example, that the discussion of this single subject (dealing with a complaint by the workers against what they thought to be undue pressure by the management for production) passed through five distinct phases or periods. Each phase or period may be designated or interpreted in terms of its relation to the total conference procedure. Thus, the first period began with a report presented by the Employee Chairman; from this point onward the Management Chairman proceeded to explain the principles guiding Management with respect to problems of this sort; in addition he challenged the Employee's assumptions; this period of the conference involved seventeen participating units, of which the Management Chairman's discourse consumed sixteen. The second phase is called "The Period of Discovery of Difficulties", and here we find a distribution of participation, although the Management Chairman contributes eight units, and Employee Representative three, and a visitor [1] four. The succeeding or third phase is called "The Period of Solution Offered by the Management Chairman", and here again we find this chairman contributing seventeen units without any additional participation by other members of the committee. In the fourth phase, "Period of Further Elaboration of Diffi-

---

[1] In this particular company visitors are frequently invited to sit with joint committees, but such visitors are invariably technicians who possess special knowledge concerning the subject under consideration. Or, they are persons who have had special and relevant experience although not members of this particular committee.

culties ", one notes another distribution in which, however, only the Employee Chairman and one other Employee Representative take part. Finally, there is a culminating phase, " The Period of Conclusion ", in which the Management Chairman, after one relevant statement of experience by an employee, formulates the policy, states the manner of disposing of this item of business, and invites the confidence of the employees.

One further reference to the chart will reveal that we have appended an additional column of interpretations under the title " Psychological."[1] In this column we have merely attempted to indicate, in terms of the phase or period, what appeared to be the dominant attitude, in so far as this attitude seemed to be a part of the purposive element in the discourse. Thus, the complete chart, that is, complete so far as we have developed this technique, includes six aspects of committee interaction, namely : (a) the number of units of participation involved, (b) the person participating, (c) the descriptive quality of each unit of participation, (d) the flow of participation from person to person, (e) a grouping of units into conference phases, or periods, together with some interpretation of

[1] The validity of these psychological categories derives frankly from inferences of language content. Since the meetings analysed were those of joint committees consisting of Management and Employee representatives, it might be feasible to postulate a set of psychological polarities ; with the aid of these, it might become a simpler task to designate the dominant attitudes for each period of the conference. We suggest, for example, such polar concepts as :

Dominance	.	. Submission
Offensive	.	. Defensive
Confidence	.	. Suspicion
Assertion	.	. Denial
Conciliation	.	. Irreconciliation

the relation of these parts to the whole, and (f) a tentative interpretation of the psychological (attitudinal) correlate of each phase or period of the discussion.

The Methodological and Psychological columns in the chart on page 195 bear directly upon the question of what is or what is not " good " conference method, and what is or is not " good " conference conduct. In our investigations we discovered that personnel officials and other industrial officers were most eager to receive enlightenment with respect to this vexing problem. So persistent were their requests that we found this to be one of the most challenging and perplexing difficulties to be encountered. In short, these persons were already so sensitized to the need for improved conference methods that they were prepared to take didactic advice whether based upon research or not. Since we made the initial assumption that we could never arrive at trustworthy facts unless our research purpose somehow and at various points coalesced with the purposes of those involved in joint committees, we could not withstand these demands entirely. But, wherever possible we allowed our material, inadequate and incomplete as it was, to do the teaching. Thus, a chart such as the above which reveals that the Management Chairman contributed forty-nine of the total of seventy-one units of participation, that no other Management Representative participated at all, and that only three of twelve Employee Representatives participated, is in itself a teaching device of unmistakable implications. This chart also reveals numerous other clues with respect to conference method, for example, it shows that the solution was presented by the Management Chairman and that his authority carried this unaltered solution through to acceptance. If the members of this committee knew this to be the characteristic method of this chairman, no wide distribution of participation could be expected.

But, the fundamental problem of " good " or " valid " conference method is one which does not belong in a volume concerned primarily with research hypotheses and techniques. The very techniques which we suggest in this volume will, we hope, furnish the kind of knowledge concerning the intricacies of interaction in committees which are needed before adequate and sound rules for conference method may be proposed. The so-called practical persons who wish so ardently to know how to " run " committees appear to reduce the problem to absurd simplicity. They overlook, for example, the fact that committee method is directly related to committee purpose. Since there are, obviously, many purposes involved in committees, there can be no single method appropriate for all purposes. A technician could, of course, advise any given industrial concern with respect to its complete system of managerial, employee and joint committees, providing he could be sure at the outset that all of the persons involved in the membership of these committees were aware of their purposes. So long as an industry, for example, utilizes joint committees, to absorb latent conflicts, to sustain morale, or to forestall trade unionism, and is frank in stating these purposes, there is an easy pathway to appropriate conference method. If, however, industries actually utilize joint-committees for true problem-solving and as an integral part of management, then the road toward sound con-

N

ference method is complex and difficult. All that can be said at present is that very few industries have recognized and stated their realistic purposes with respect to joint committees and consequently no one can suggest to them the " best " conference method.

A Simpler Form of Charting.

Those who may wish to experiment with the charting of committee meetings but who are not prepared to utilize the complex system of categories, or units of participation, suggested above, may find use for a more elementary form. Instead of separating the participation into units consisting of single statements and queries, a more generalized unit may be utilized. In this case, a person's total and continuous discourse for any given participation would be used as the unit ; this may be described in one or more phrases and in terms of its main purport. Although less explicit and more subjective in character, this device of charting possesses the advantage of simplicity. In this form of chart the time element must be taken into account by spreading the units over a relatively larger space. An illustration of a more simplified form of charting is presented on the following page.

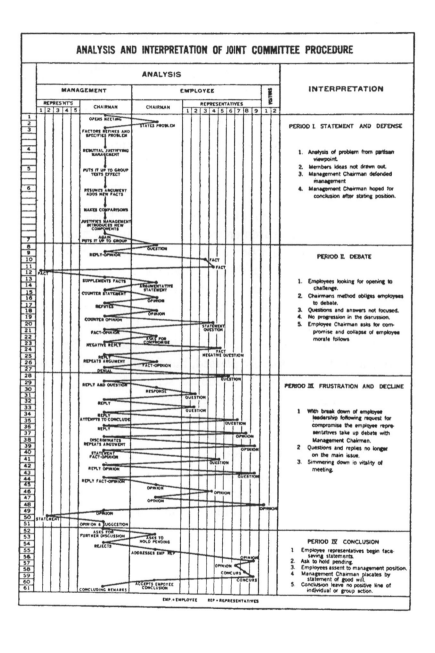

CHAPTER XIV

THE PLACE OF STATISTICAL DEVICES
IN PSYCHO-SOCIAL RESEARCH

(Basic Form : Person-to-Record Situation)

REALISTIC social control, without the slightest doubt, depends upon measurement. But, what kind of measurement ? It is at this point that social scientists confront their most difficult problem. There are some who are wholly impatient with the refinement of categories and with processes ; they wish to count whatever seems objective and simple. If only a sufficient quantity of facts may be gathered and correlated, these investigators appear to be, not merely pleased, but assured of the future utility of their work. Graduate schools, governmental departments, and business establishments continue to accumulate statistical enumerations of this simple variety, but the percentage which becomes actually usable for social control is lamentably small. Indeed, an accounting of the sums of money already spent and now being spent on quantitative researches which cannot possibly bear any practical relation to human affairs might take on the proportions of a public scandal.[1] In so far as the social

[1] " The mere accumulation of measurements, of data, of facts (which may not really be facts after all) may be a worthless expenditure of time, energy, and money. To be sure, there are problems which are up to the present time susceptible of study only by the inductive method ; but it is of the very essence of science that the investigator have an idea, though he hold ever so lightly to it."—*Universities*, by Abraham Flexner, p. 127.

sciences are concerned, there appear to be sufficient reasons for believing that the problem of measurement needs to be re-examined. The discipline of these sciences promises to produce, not thinkers and scholars, but skilled manipulators of mathematical formulæ. Whether the final results of statistical devices are important or not seems to matter very little so long as these may be regarded as " statistically valid." This claim for statistical validity has been pushed so far in the direction of absurdity that even the statisticians are beginning to profess misgivings.

The Rôle of Statistics in the Whole of Method.

Critical readers will have observed that our discussion of research techniques began with those which are usually considered less objective, and that we have gradually moved toward those in which the objective element reveals an increment. This sequence should not betray the reader : as one advances toward the more objective techniques one also utilizes more of abstraction. Science is most certain when most abstract. When the units have been thoroughly abstracted, when the cluttering fragments of direct experience have dropped by the wayside, then ideas seem " pure " and unmixed. Thus, mathematics may serve as the ultimate example of abstraction, and it is because of its " pureness " that social scientists have, no doubt, hurried toward its methods.[1] In moving from Interviewing to Statistics we have, therefore, been aware of the fact that our units have

---

[1] Astronomy is, perhaps, the most accurate of the sciences, and also the farthest removed from sensuous human experience.

become increasingly artificial. Interviewing, so to speak, catches life on the wing ; what the interviewer sees is mixed, scrambled, and confused but possesses the quality of moving experience. In like manner, the Direct Observation of a committee in session provides the investigator with a " rough slice " of reality. Participant Observing and Case Analysis involve increasing increments of abstraction until at last we come to the highest level of abstraction, namely, Statistics.

Statistical Records as Found in Industries.

Wherever joint committees exist in modern industries it happens that considerable time and money is spent on keeping records. Minutes of all meetings are recorded, copies made and distributed. A statistician is employed to select certain items from these minutes and he constructs tables and charts. Where records of committee meetings were reduced to enumerative categories we found that facts of the following varieties were recorded :

(*a*) Number of committee meetings held per year ;

(*b*) Number of management representatives involved ;

(*c*) Number of employee representatives involved ;

(*d*) Age of participants ;

(*e*) Length of service of participants ;

(*f*) Subjects discussed (according to private and non-analytical categories) ;

(*g*) Kinds of settlements reached ;

(*h*) Decisions reached in favour of either management or employees.

It will be noted that the first five of these categories represent simple and obvious facts, units of persons or time. Such facts are, obviously, useful to management as a part of its complete personnel record, but have very little significance for research. The last three items, however, are representative of the functional aspects of committees and provide a real clue for research.

Statistics as Applied to Significant Aspects of Committee Process.

Social facts, then, seem to offer a choice between those of a concrete physical existence on the one hand and of an intangible psychic quality on the other. But it is precisely this psychic quality which is the stuff of social reality.

In the beginning we entertained a somewhat simplified conception of the measurable features of committee functioning. We sought answers to three major queries, namely:

(1) What problem is the committee confronting? (Problem, or Subject-matter)

(2) What procedure of conferencing is the committee following? (Process)

(3) What kinds of results does the committee achieve? (Conclusion)

We believed that simple correlations might be made with the use of these categories. For example, does the committee achieve one kind of result with a specific kind of procedure? Does the committee utilize the same procedure for all types of problems? If the reader will now refer to Chapter V on *Interaction*, he will see to what extent we have refined the " process " category, and it now becomes necessary to indicate how, through a similar procedure of refinements, we have dealt with the problem of subject-matter, or committee business.

An Inductive-Deductive Device for Deriving Subject-matter Categories.

What kinds of problems do joint committees in industry discuss ? It appears as a simple task to designate the subjects discussed at any given meeting, but once one begins to classify these random topics, difficulties of many sorts arise. If an official in charge of joint committees is asked what the committees in his company discuss, the response is immediate ; he replies, " They discuss wages, hours, and working conditions." This simple answer is also reflected in the statistical records kept by the various companies. But closer inspection soon reveals that these categories simply " grew " in industrial parlance and that very little attention has been given to their ampli-fication and clarification. One discovers ambiguities, inconsistencies, and important omissions. When, for example, a new type or problem is recognized it is simply subsumed under one or the other of these traditional categories. In short, these " frozen terms " as found in industrial records could not be utilized as the basis for an accurate interpretation of what transpires in joint com-mittees. Recognizing this difficulty, we were then, as research agents, compelled to ask two questions, namely : Would a standardized set of subject-matter categories be useful to us as investigators, and to those persons in industries responsible for the recording and analysing of committee data ? Second : By what processes could a standardized set of categories be derived ? The first question was readily answered : we agreed that a more significant and standard set of categories would supply us with fresh meanings and would be, for our purposes, more useful than the private and more or less accidental classifications found in the records. The second query was not so easily answered.

Steps Leading Toward a Classification of Subject-matter.

All categories, and all classifications, no matter how simple, are abstractions. Any departure from the raw sense data of experience, from the living situation, involves an abstract procedure. On the other hand, the total situation can never be wholly apprehended, not to say comprehended : our perceptual capacities are not able to register the many-sided actuality of the living present. What transpires after the event, to use Cassirer's [1] term, is construction, or reconstruction, reformulation, and rearrangement according to habitual and rationalized patterns. " In our exploration of the external world," says Ritchie,[2] " we have to reject or neglect a very large part of what is given in experience in order to be able to

[1] " But genuine, theoretically guided induction is never satisfied merely with establishing facts as given. It replaces the factual co-existence of sensuous data by another kind of connection, which indeed seems poorer in elements when considered purely materially, but which can be more clearly surveyed according to the principle of construction. Every experiment we institute, and on which we base our inductive inferences, works in this direction. The real object of scientific investigation is never the raw material of sensuous perception ; in place of this science substitute a system of conditions constructed and defined by itself."—E. Cassirer, *Substance, Function and Einstein's Theory of Relativity*, p. 253.

[2] *Scientific Method*, by A. D. Ritchie, pp. 199–200.

make use of the remainder. What we do make use of has to be treated by very elaborate processes before the raw material of experience is converted into the finished product of scientific theory. When the process is all over, it is very difficult to see the connection between what we started with and what we finish with. The world of immediate experience is an affair of blurred and fluctuating outlines of meaningless variegation, it is full of loose ends, of vague relations to something outside its immediate content. Out of this we construct something neat and tidy, something compact and rounded off. Yet we are compelled to believe that the last is somehow a true reflection of the first. It may be a distorted reflection, but the distortion goes by rule, so that the image is veridical even if it is not veritable." This description of the pathway between raw experience and refined science represents accurately the procedure which was followed in the present case : we began with the raw data of committee meetings as transcribed in the records ; these we have sifted and winnowed and examined until at last we have arrived at a manageable set of categories which, we believe, denote with some degree of accuracy the subject-matter of joint committees in industry. We now proceed to describe the pathway along which we have travelled.

An artificial classification is one based upon predetermined, *a priori* purpose. An investigator might wish to know, for example, how many items in a given total of committee sessions were devoted to wages ; he would then proceed to extract from the data, without critical examination, all those items which were either representative of wages or not-wages. His purpose would, then, predetermine the classification. A procedure of this sort is, of course, justifiable, especially in cases where the investigator is thoroughly familiar with the nature of the data. It proceeds, however, from a subjective base, and is, therefore, susceptible to all the dangers inherent in a situation in which specific purposes guide specific inquiries. Most investigators recognize the amazing ease with which one may eliminate, or fail to recognize, facts which do not fit *a priori* classifications.

A natural classification is one which is derived from inductions flowing from examination of the data. It begins by placing together things (items) which are identical or alike. The decision concerning that which is alike and that which is different cannot be reached by methods which are purely inductive. (Perhaps, the use of words in itself violates pure inductive method.) *Likeness*, according to Whewell, is not established by definition but by properties, since " before we can attend to several things as like or unlike, we must be able to apprehend each of these by itself as one thing. This unity," he continues, " is given by the mind itself ; the condition of unity of an object is that assertions concerning it shall be possible."[1] One must be able, that is, to apply many verbs to one substantive. Whewell maintains, however, that in setting up a natural classification as, for example, in plants, a general knowledge of the subject is necessary and that " other ideas must be called into action as well as the idea of likeness." A natural classification based upon essential likeness and difference must not be presumed to be exclusive of all other classifications, even

[1] *The History of Scientific Ideas*, by William Whewell, p. 95.

other natural ones. Natural classifications may vary with respect to general, but never with respect to specific, purposes and conveniences.[1]

Whewell, in maintaining that likeness can only be determined by properties and not by definition, appears to limit the adaptability of natural classifications to those properties which are measurable. In the case of psycho-social phenomena it is precisely the most important of all properties and qualities which escapes measurement. In analysing the subjects coming before joint committees, one is dealing, not with *things*, but rather with propositions. It appears, then, that in studies of this sort discriminations between likeness and difference cannot be based upon accurate measurement either of things or properties. Before proceeding, therefore, we must be more specific with respect to the *whatness* of these subjects appearing as items of business in committee meetings.

For present purposes it may be assumed that there are three general classes of phenomena to be observed in the universe, namely, *objects*, *events*, and *representations of objects or events* (thoughts).

This conception may be diagramed as follows :

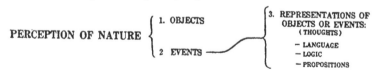

PERCEPTION OF NATURE { 1. OBJECTS / 2 EVENTS — { 3. REPRESENTATIONS OF OBJECTS OR EVENTS: (THOUGHTS) — LANGUAGE — LOGIC — PROPOSITIONS

---

[1] " Misled, as we shall see, by the problem of classification in the natural sciences, philosophers often seem to think that in each subject there must be one essentially natural classification which is to be selected to the exclusion of the other. This erroneous notion probably proceeds also in part from the limited powers of thought and inconvenient mechanical conditions under which we labour."—*Principles of Science*, 1874 ed., p. 345, Stanley Jevons.

The subject-matter of a committee's deliberations appears initially, not as object, but as event. The investigator's observation is not, however, of the event but of a representation of the event found in written, recorded language. Using this diagram as the skeletal background for classifications, it may be said that :

1. *Objects* may be classified according to measurements ; the properties involved may also be classified by objective measurements.

2. *Events* are subject to space-time measurement, but complete and accurate denotation and description on the part of the observer is impossible ; inference of one sort or another must always be invoked in defining the event.

3. *Representations*, or symbols of objects and events, appear to us in language forms. In the case of the joint committee, for example, we discover what event has transpired, or more specifically, what subject was deliberated upon, by reading the record of the meeting. But, the language form, or mode, which represents the event is not the chief consideration ; our aim is to discover, beyond this form, beyond this representation, a *what* which has its incidence not in language but in the operation of a given industry.

Subjects are presented to the committee, either in written or oral form ; the essential deposit of this event is a proposition.[1] But, it is always a proposition *about*

[1] " A verbal statement is assumed to be the expression of a proposition ; this assumption implies that there is a genuine difference between the statement as a form of words and the proposition which

something, representative of an essential idea. And, it is *something about* which needs to be registered in categories of likeness and sameness. Our problem has now been located in the field of logic ; we are hence prepared to describe our verbal-logic events, or their representations, by definition and not by measurement.

Before proceeding, however, it may be advisable to state the general criteria used as tests for categories of this sort. We have assumed that a valid set of categories depicting the subject discussed in joint committees would :

1. Be qualitatively consistent ;
2. Admit of sharp definition ;
3. Be sufficiently interrelated and indeterminate to allow for degrees of combination and re-combination ;
4. Be sufficiently numerous to be comprehensive and still few enough in number to be manageable, and if necessary to be suitable for statistical tabulations and correlations.

In addition to these primary criteria, we also assumed that it would be desirable, if possible, to arrive at a final set of categories of subject-matter which would :

(*a*) Be applicable to all joint committees in all industries;
(*b*) Allow for comparisons between various committees at various periods of time ;
(*c*) Be consistent with and form a definite part of a set of categories to cover the whole of industry.

is thereby stated. The difference is analogous to the difference between symbols and their meanings. A proposition is what the classical tradition called an idea, a significant form ; and a verbal statement, if it is significant, is significant by reference to ideas."—*Dialectic*, by Mortimer Adler, p. 143.

Inductive and Deductive Methods Conjoined.

The psychological factors which intrude themselves into the process of forming logical concepts should be initially recognized. There is no pure method of thought. Logic formalizes thought but it does not wholly succeed in eliminating wish and purpose. And, in so far as thinking is performed through the use of language, each idea will be found to consist of a central core of relatively realistic content, plus a periphery of subjective accumulations. Induction and deduction are popularly presumed to be opposite methods of reasoning, but closer scrutiny invariably reveals the fact that these two modes of thought are mixed, intertwined. Or, as Bogoslovsky states, " The old logic differentiated definitely between them. Deduction was considered as an application of the general principle to a particular case and induction as the opposite process of constructing a general rule from particular instances. As the movements run in quite opposite directions, they were even thought to be mutually exclusive for any single operation of reasoning. But, as a matter of fact, we always have, in any act of thought, both deduction and induction, only under certain conditions we have the inductive element predominant, in other circumstances the deductive tendency prevailing."[1]

The data, consisting as it does of records of past meetings, represents a verbal summary of events. In each instance the investigator must ask, " What were these persons talking about ? " The " *what* " in recorded data becomes the basic unit in classification, and until

[1] *The Technique of Controversy*, pp. 104–105.

this "*whatness*" has been clarified it is useless to apply quantitative methods of analysis.[1] The "*whatness*" of the record cannot be measured; it can only be reasoned about. All that can be done to make this procedure objective is to distinguish between likeness and difference, but even here non-objective means are utilized; likeness and difference are properties, not so much of the objects or events in themselves as of the mind of the observer. At every point of discrimination between likeness and difference the observer's psychological hinterland, the source of all general propositions, intrudes itself as part of his judgment.[2] Thus, when the inductive process is

[1] A similar problem of categories was confronted in an analogous study of newspaper content. (*The Country Newspaper* : Willey.) This investigator's task was to designate each article according to some subject-matter category. (See also *News and the Newspaper*, by Kingsbury, Hart and Clark, *The New Republic*, October 8, 1930.) The "*whatness*" of these newspaper articles, as well as the "*whatness*" of committee minutes becomes, then, the chief element in classification.

[2] "The chief points of postulate theory are that no demonstration can be made except in terms of some propositions which are not demonstrated, though not necessarily not demonstrable ; that such undemonstrated propositions, usually called postulates, are taken as true without proof ; that the process of definition requires the acceptation of certain terms as undefinable in any given set of definitions ; that such indefinables are taken as having precise meaning though undefined ; that, in short, any logical demonstration whether called a doctrine or a system, depends in logical origin upon a set of primitives—postulates, definitions, and indefinables—and that within any given system or doctrine, these primitives are themselves not submitted to the processes of demonstration.

"These primitives, then, are non-rational elements in the process of thinking and this is equally so whether that thinking be inductive or deductive, demonstrative or argumentative. They are usually not considered to be absolute ; that is, there is no one set of primitives obligatory upon all thinking, and necessary to every system. Postulates and definitions are the logical equivalents of what the psychologist calls prejudices and wilful thinking. They are chosen or selected, rather than intellectually obligatory and rationally unavoidable. The most

begun it already contains a deductive element, namely, the observer's unconscious, or half-conscious background of assimilated concepts ; without these he cannot make discriminations. The inductive process, then, may be said always to begin with the general, that which is in the mind of the reasoner ; it then deals with the particular, but in the end returns to the general, thus :

From the *General :* Unconscious psychological concepts.

To *Particular :* Object of attention.

To *General :* Conscious, logical concepts.

If, then, " induction remains at all, which is a difficult question, it will remain merely as one of the principles according to which deductions are effected."[1] Final categories, if these result from rigorous analysis, will be generalized abstractions. The degree of generalization and abstraction possible in any given case will be determined by the nature of the data, and the investigator's wishes.[2] This interrelated use of inductive and deductive methods may now be set forth in terms of specific stages. The total process of deriving appropriate categories, beginning with the event and ending with concepts suitable for research purposes, comprises seven separate steps ; we are here excluding the first two steps, namely, noting the event and recording it verbally, since these

general name for such elements is ' *intuitive propositions,*' when intuition is taken to mean not the manner in which we know a true proposition but the manner in which we know a proposition taken as true."— *Dialectic,* by Mortimer Adler, pp. 14–15.

[1] *Scientific Method in Philosophy,* by Bertrand Russell, p. 34.

[2] For a suggestive treatment of this and the previous discussion on psychological and logical concepts, see I. Miller, *The Psychology of Thinking,* Chapters 15–19.

o

occurred before research was initiated. Specifically stated, the five stages through which the material was passed in deriving subject-matter categories were :

1. *Examination of the Material:* Type-written minutes of committee meetings, usually in summary and not verbatim form, were available. The investigators were already familiar with this material, having utilized it for a variety of other purposes over a period of a year or more. In the present examination, however, attention was directed at one aspect only, namely, the discovery of *what* was discussed in each item presented. At this stage, verb-noun combinations or descriptive statements lifted from the total context, and registered. This procedure, as will be seen, constitutes a sort of " fixing-bath " in which subjects are caught in their most elemental state.

2. *Aggregation of the Subject Items :* The descriptive statements are assembled so that scrutiny is possible to aid in the formation of groups. This is the first formative stage in the inductive-deductive process. They are perceived as a mass of data in the rough without identifying elements of likeness and difference.

3. *Classification of the Subject Items by Placement in Primary Groups according to Likeness :* Likeness, in this case, meant identity wherever identity was obvious, but it also meant correspondence or consimilarity with respect to problem-context. For example, if the members of the committee discuss whether wages shall be paid by bank draft or cash, they are not discussing wages *per se*, but rather methods of payment : the problem-

context, then, is methods-of-payment and not wages. In each case, the question was asked, Is likeness here greater than difference ? If difference is greater than likeness, a new classificatory group needs to be formed. (*Note.*—There is, patently, a great deal of subjectivity involved in these choices between likeness and difference ; the investigator's unconscious wishes, even his positive or negative feeling about words, enters and colours his choice. For this reason, this procedure is more valid when used by more than one person, that is, by two or more persons correcting each other's judgments during the process. Comparison of the various items in the groups can best be facilitated by following some procedure such as this :

(*a*) State the points wherein the items are related ;

(*b*) State the salient points wherein the items are different.

(*c*) If the points of likeness are more important than the points of difference, give a generalized statement of these points of likeness that will serve for identifying the group.)

4. *The Abstraction of Titles for Groups of Subject Items :* The process of abstraction is similar to that of comparison in that it consists of a further formation of groups. But in this instance it is a grouping of groups. The subordinate groupings are recombined into a larger whole on the basis of their essential common qualities. The point of departure for determining these essential common qualities is in the psychological concepts on which the study is based, that is, the

background knowledge of the subject-matter plus the purpose of the investigator to construct a relevant set of categories. Abstraction proper is a decantation of the essential, common qualities of the elements represented in the groups and a holding of them up for separate consideration. When this has been done for the whole of the data, a number of these abstractions remain which should be the true connotation of all data. The use of terms in this and the following state is subject to particular hazards. Specific, unambiguous meanings are difficult to determine. Particular care must be exercised in maintaining a common co-ordinate level in the abstractions.

5. *The Generalization of Subject-matter Terms :* The previous stage of abstraction should give a suitable set of concepts for dealing with the massed data. For purposes of wider usage, however, one more step toward the intensive is important. This last or generalization stage is valuable in showing the possible relations of these subjects to a larger body of data that deal with industry as a whole and not merely with such items as come under consideration in an employee representation plan. Subject categories that are valid for employee representation must also be valid for industry in general. The test for validity is to see if these final generalizations fit co-ordinately and subordinately into such a broader set of categories. This final step in abstraction involves the use of knowledge plus insight. Terms of this nature must, to some degree at least, be invented. The process is similar to that of the archæologist who must construct a complete pattern, an entire pot from a few fragments.

How successful the present investigators have been in devising final categories is still to be determined ; only a wide usage of these categories will indicate whether or not they convey accurate meanings.

By using a random selection of five hundred items presented in committees of two large industries the following result was obtained : [1]

Classification or Primary Grouping	Abstraction or Secondary Grouping	Generalization or Final Grouping
(Classifying of items)	(Classifying of groups)	
Methods of work. Methods of dealing with customer. Suggestions to management on process. Rules for work. Tools and equipment. Elimination of dangers and annoyances.	Ways and means of doing work. Physical surroundings of the job.	PERFORMING.
Qualifications for the job. Classification of the job. Preparation and training for job. Responsibility added to job. Assistance needed on job. Age limit for retiring. Surplus and deficit of working force. Promotions, demotions, transfers, discipline. Temporary separation from the pay-roll. Hours of work, schedules of overtime. Leaves of absence without pay.	Standardization of job. Adjustment of personnel in number, status and time.	REGULATING.

[1] The first and second stages are omitted for obvious reason of bulk.

Classification or Primary Grouping	Abstraction or Secondary Grouping	Generalization or Final Grouping
Holidays. Vacations. Civic and military service.	Pay for time absent from work by permission.	
Rates for individuals and groups. Basis for payment. Defining rates.	Establishment and maintenance of rates.	
Sale of company stock Sale of company goods. Sale of insurance. Concessions on hospital fees. Concessions on housing rental.	Goods, services and economics for employees.	REWARDING.
Pensions. Death benefits. Sickness benefits.	Compensation for sickness, accidents and long service.	
Facilities for employee purchases. Facilities for employee saving. Facilities for employee transportation. Facilities for health, medical and dental service. Safety and accident prevention. Method, time, period of wage payment. Food service. Lockers and bath facilities.	Conveniences and privileges and facilities for employees.	ENVIRONING.
Goodwill, gratitude, tribute and condolence. Employee Representation Plan and its committees.	Group expressions and activities.	

Miscellaneous.

Beginning, then, with five hundred random items of business performed by joint committees in three representative industries as stated in the record, we ended the inductive-deductive procedure when we had arrived at four major categories which seemed to us sufficiently abstract to be usable as designations for all types of committee subject-matter. Whether these categories are broad enough to be applicable in all industries and for all types of joint committees can only be determined by further experimentation. Our main objective was to derive such categories as might be useful for statistical purposes. The subject-matter of joint committees in industry, then, falls into a classification of four terms, namely, (1) *Performing work*, (2) *Regulating work and conditions of work*, (3) *Rewarding for work done or to be done*, and (4) *Environing, including psychological (morale) as well as physical conditions under which work is performed*. Philosophically, these categories have wide usage, but for statistical purposes within any given industry the thirteen sub-categories need to be used because of their specific character.

An Abstract Formula Suitable for Statistical Purposes.

The foregoing account of the theory and practice of deriving categories represents a laborious procedure through which we have purposely taken the reader ; our aim has been, not merely to indicate how we arrived at the place of selecting four major categories suitable for research but also to emphasize the necessity of utilizing modern logic in the various stages of research. Not many research students who have been " bitten " by the current fashion of " counting " will be prepared to submit themselves to logical necessities of this sort, but we believe that the emphasis should be made, nevertheless. In any case, we may now eliminate considerable detail from the description of the remaining phases of our statistical formula. Suffice it to say that we concluded that simple descriptive categories were not suitable for statistical purposes and that we needed abstract categories, terms which might be used to denote the psycho-social process. The S–O–R formula developed in Chapter V appeared to furnish the clue for such categories, and we have therefore assumed that the dynamics of joint committee processes might be measured in terms of Stimulus, Organization, and Response. Our next task was to provide these categories with meaningful content as related to committees. The joint committee as function or process may, then, be reduced to quantitative bases if the following facts are tabulated :

A. *Stimulus :*

    1. Subject-matter area. (See pages 213 and 214 for details.)

    2. The manner of introducing the subject :

        (*a*) Simple : matter-of-fact, oral pronouncement or written announcement ;

        (*b*) Amplified : simple statement or reading plus explanation or introduction of supporting facts ;

        (*c*) Weighted : may be either simple or amplified but with an additional element of argument intended to influence or condition the attitudes of conferees.

3. Language mode used in introducing subject :
   (*a*) Written ;
   (*b*) Oral.

B. *Organization :*

  1. Implicit individual consideration ; unspoken.
  2. Explicit individual consideration ; spoken :
     (*a*) Individual to individual ; single ;
     (*b*) Individual to individual ; recurrent.
  3. Explicit collective consideration :
     (*a*) Employee representatives only ;
     (*b*) Management representatives only ;
     (*c*) Both employee and management represen-
     tatives.

C. *Response :* [1]

  1. Implicit, non-overt or tacit conclusion.
  2. Explicit, overt conclusion :
     (*a*) Acceptance of proposal, suggestion, or state-
     ment :
        (i) Provisional ;
        (ii) Tentative (with allowance for recon-
        sideration) ;
        (iii) Apparently complete.
     (*b*) Delegation of responsibility to person or
     persons who are members of the joint
     committee :
        (i) To management in general ;
        (ii) To specific management person ;

---

[1] As now used for statistical purposes, this term " response " may be thought of as including the meanings of " result," " consummation," or " emergence."

    (iii) To employees in general ;

    (iv) To specific employee ;

    (v) To a special committee.

(c) Assumption of responsibility by person or persons who are members of the joint committee :

    (i) By management chairman ;

    (ii) By management in general ;

    (iii) By employees in general ;

    (iv) By specific employee ;

    (v) By a special committee.

(d) Rejection of proposal, suggestion, or statement.

(e) Withdrawal of proposal, suggestion, or statement.

(f) Conclusion deferred :

    (i) For further information from Management, employee, both, jointly, et cetera.

    (ii) For investigation by management, employees, both (separately), joint committee, et cetera.

    (iii) For further authority.

    (iv) For other reasons.

(g) Referred to person or persons not members of the joint committee, but to be reported back to the joint committee :

    (i) To management ;

    (ii) To employee, or employees ;

(iii) To a committee :
— higher in jurisdiction ;
— lower in jurisdiction ;
— special.

(iv) Other.

If the above classification of categories were now placed across the top of a sheet of paper, with each item of business listed in the left-hand column, statistical tabulations could be made as follows :

Item of Business	Stimulus									Organization					Response								
	1				2			3		1		2		3	1	2							
	a	b	c	d	a	b	c	a	b	a	b	a	b	c		a	b	c	d	e	f	g	
1.																							
2.																							
3.																							
4.																							
5.																							

It will be noted that the above list of categories does not include the term " purpose." It would be useful, obviously, to know at the point of stimulation precisely what purpose the introducer of an item of business had in mind. Such purpose is discoverable in some instances but is, on the whole, concealed and cannot, therefore, be utilized quantitatively.

Each item would then be checked as far as it carried across the sheet. Thus, a glance would indicate the subject, the manner of introduction, the language mode used in introducing subject (S) ; the nature of the organization preliminary to response (O) ; and, finally, the implicit or explicit disposition of the item (R). Correlations might then be made between all of the categories checked for each item. By showing the percentage of the items of business, going only as far as S, the research agent may determine to what extent the committees are being utilized for informative or routine procedures. If he tabulates the numbers which go only as far as O, he may determine the amount of simple, non-controversial, and non-consummatory discussion engaging the time of such committees. Finally, by tabulating those which go all the way to R, he may determine by ratios and correlations the extent to which items of discussion reach a formal conclusion.

A Sample of One Hundred Joint Committee Items Treated Statistically :

STIMULUS :

Subject-matter of discussion :

Ways and means of doing work . .	34
Physical Surroundings of the job . .	2
Standardization of the job . . .	0
Adjustment of Personnel in number, status, and time	6
Pay for time absent from work by permission	1
Carry forward .	43

Brought forward . 43
Establishment and maintenance of rates
    of pay 0
Goods, services and economics for em-
    ployees 3
Compensation for sickness, accidents,
    and long service 0
Conveniences, privileges and facilities
    for employees 30
Group expressions and activities . . 19
Miscellaneous 5
                   Total . —— 100

Language Mode used in Introducing subject :
Oral 88
Written 12
                   Total . ——100

Method of introducing the subject :
Simple 67
Amplified 16
Weighted 17
                   Total . —— 100

ORGANIZATION :
Implicit, individual consideration ; unspoken 40
Explicit, individual ; spoken :
    Single, individual to individual . . 32
    Single, recurrent 1
Explicit collective consideration :
    Employee representatives only . . 11
    Management representatives only . . 2
            Carry forward . 86

Brought forward . 86

Both management and employee representatives 14

Total . —— 100

RESPONSE :

(Total of items receiving explicit organization) . 60

Implicit, non-overt response or conclusion 10

Explicit, overt conclusion :

Acceptance of proposal, suggestion, or statement:

Provisional 0

Tentative 0

Apparently complete . . . 13

Total . —— 13

Delegation of responsibility to members of committee :

To management generally . 1

To specific management person . 9

To employees generally . . 0

To specific employee . . 0

Total . —— 10

Assumption of responsibility by
members of committee :

Management person generally . 0

Management persons specifically 9

Employees generally . . 0

Employees specifically . . 1

Total . —— 10

Rejection of proposal, suggestion of statement 0

Carry forward . 43

Brought forward . 43

Withdrawal of proposal, suggestion or

statement I

Conclusions deferred :

For further information :

From management . . 0
From employees . . . 2
From both (independently) . I
From both jointly . . 0
Other I

Total . —— 4

For investigation :

By management . . . 2
By employees . . . 0
By both (independently) . 0
By both jointly . . . 0

Total . —— 2

For authority 0
For other reason I

Conclusions referred outside committee :

To management . . . 9
To employees . . . 0
To committees . . . 0

—— 9

Total of items concluded . . . —— 60

Other relevant statistical data :

Items representing old business . . . 17
Items representing new business . . . 83

Total . —— 100

Items introduced by management representatives 43
Items introduced by employee representatives 57

Total . —— 100

Summary.

The items of committee business dealt with above, one hundred in number, were selected at random from the minutes of previous meetings and have been used, not to prove anything by way of research results, but merely to illustrate how the S–O–R formula might become the basis for statistical measurement. Under the major category " S " we find that 34 per cent of the items concerned specifically ways and means of performing work, 30 per cent had to do with conveniences, privileges, and facilities for employees, 19 per cent were items dealing with employee representation itself and with its committees ; the remaining 17 per cent of items represented scattering subjects such as physical surroundings, payment for time absent from work, et cetera. As a part of stimulus, we may note that 88 per cent of the items were introduced orally, while 12 per cent arose from written reports or references. Sixty-seven of the total of one hundred items were brought before the committees by means of simple statements or questions.

The " O " column, or organization of response, reveals considerably more of the essence of committee process, since we note at once that 40 per cent of the items coming before the committees receive no overt consideration of any sort ; these items were simply presented and were not discussed. Of the remaining 60 per cent, more than one half received consideration only by two persons and not by the group as a whole. Thus, of the total of one hundred items only 27, or slightly more than one-fourth, were treated collectively, that is, by the employee representatives and the management chairman ; only 14 of the total received consideration by employees and management representatives other than the chairman.

Reviewing the treatment of the total one hundred cases, we discover that 40 per cent stopped at " S " or stimulus ; these items were presented to the group as information, suggestion, or advice and elicited no response. Of the remaining sixty items, fifty reached the stage of explicit conclusion ; thirteen of these were suggestions or proposals which the groups accepted, twenty were disposed of by delegating responsibility, and action on sixteen was delayed because the final conclusion was referred to other committees or authorities. This brief summary gives some insight into the kind of factual material which might be derived from a statistical study of such committees. As a test of the adequacy of committees, this technique would need to be carried to the stage of correlations. At this point the statistical technique would need to be brought into relation with case analysis ; when, for example, a committee disposes of an item by reference to another authority, this reference would hereafter need to be followed until an ultimate conclusion of some sort had been reached.

P

POSTSCRIPT

Experimentation with research techniques in the social sciences needs to be carried to still a further level. What is needed is a demonstration of the conjoint use of all techniques in relation to a single problem or situation. (A combined approach of this sort might, of course, include techniques not discussed in this volume, for example, the questionnaire.) Each technique will presumably reveal a different quality of fact ; moreover, each separate technique may reveal a varying quality of fact when used by different investigators. The statistician may not be an adept at interviewing, and the person who is proficient in observing may lack the skills necessary for charting. But, if six investigators, all attempting to study a single situation in terms of an accepted set of analytical categories, were to function co-operatively, each separate skill would supplement the other and the net result would be a set of facts and interpretations immediately usable for purposes of social change. Dynamic social research is based upon the assumption that fact-finding should lead to action. Its major premise is that meaningful social action based upon knowledge will follow when social research is founded upon an inclusive epistemology and an experimental logic, that is, when its facts fall into a relativistic scale which bears some resemblance to life itself.

INDEX OF PROPER NAMES

INDEX OF SUBJECTS